Pedagogies for Pharmacy Curricula

Isabel Vitória Figueiredo
University of Coimbra, Portugal

Afonso Miguel Cavaco
University of Lisbon, Portugal

A volume in the Advances in Medical Education, Research, and Ethics (AMERE) Book Series

IGI Global
PUBLISHER of TIMELY KNOWLEDGE

Published in the United States of America by
IGI Global
Medical Information Science Reference (an imprint of IGI Global)
701 E. Chocolate Avenue
Hershey PA, USA 17033
Tel: 717-533-8845
Fax: 717-533-8661
E-mail: cust@igi-global.com
Web site: http://www.igi-global.com

Library of Congress Cataloging-in-Publication Data

Names: Figueiredo, Isabel Vitória, 1964- editor. | Cavaco, Afonso Miguel, 1966- editor.
Title: Pedagogies for pharmacy curricula / Isabel Vitória Figueiredo and Afonso Miguel Cavaco, editors.
Description: Hershey, PA : Medical Information Science Reference, [2021] | Includes bibliographical references and index. | Summary: "This book examines pedagogic methodologies on the scope of pharmaceutical care in pharmacy curricula"-- Provided by publisher.
Identifiers: LCCN 2020003264 (print) | LCCN 2020003265 (ebook) | ISBN 9781799844860 (hardcover) | ISBN 9781799844877 (ebook)
Subjects: LCSH: Pharmacy--Study and teaching.
Classification: LCC RS101 .P43 2021 (print) | LCC RS101 (ebook) | DDC 615.1076--dc23
LC record available at https://lccn.loc.gov/2020003264
LC ebook record available at https://lccn.loc.gov/2020003265

This book is published in the IGI Global book series Advances in Medical Education, Research, and Ethics (AMERE) (ISSN: 2475-6601; eISSN: 2475-661X)

British Cataloguing in Publication Data
A Cataloguing in Publication record for this book is available from the British Library.

Advances in Medical Education, Research, and Ethics (AMERE) Book Series

ISSN:2475-6601
EISSN:2475-661X

MISSION

Humans are living longer now than ever as a result of advances in the medical field. Having the tools available to train knowledgeable and ethical future generations of doctors and medical researchers is essential to continuing to advance our understanding of the human body and develop new ways of treating and curing sickness and disease.

The **Advances in Medical Education, Research, and Ethics (AMERE)** book series highlights publications pertaining to advancements in pedagogical practice for developing future healthcare professionals, research methods, and advancements in the medical field, as well as moral behavior and practice of healthcare professionals, students, and researchers. Featuring research-based book publications that are highly relevant to the healthcare community, this series is ideally designed for library inclusion at medical universities and research institutions as well as personal use by medical professionals, researchers, and upper-level students entering the field.

COVERAGE

- Clinical Research
- Conflicts of Interest
- Ethics in Medicine
- Healthcare Pedagogy
- Medical Curricula
- Medical Simulation
- Patient Data
- Professional Development
- Research Methods
- Scientific Misconduct

IGI Global is currently accepting manuscripts for publication within this series. To submit a proposal for a volume in this series, please contact our Acquisition Editors at Acquisitions@igi-global.com or visit: http://www.igi-global.com/publish/.

The Advances in Medical Education, Research, and Ethics (AMERE) Book Series (ISSN 2475-6601) is published by IGI Global, 701 E. Chocolate Avenue, Hershey, PA 17033-1240, USA, www.igi-global.com. This series is composed of titles available for purchase individually; each title is edited to be contextually exclusive from any other title within the series. For pricing and ordering information please visit http://www.igi-global.com/book-series/advances-medical-education-research-ethics/132365. Postmaster: Send all address changes to above address.

Titles in this Series

For a list of additional titles in this series, please visit:
http://www.igi-global.com/book-series/advances-medical-education-research-ethics/132365

Cases on Instructional Design and Performance Outcomes in Medical Edcation
Jill Stefaniak (University of Georgia, USA)
Medical Information Science Reference • © 2020 • 330pp • H/C (ISBN: 9781799850922) • US $265.00

Exploring Best Child Development Practices in Contemporary ociety
Nava R. Silton (Marymount Manhattan College, USA)
Medical Information Science Reference • © 2020 • 305pp • H/C (ISBN: 9781799829409) • US $245.00

Building a Patient-Centered Interprofessional Education Program
Steven D. Waldman (University of Missouri-Kansas City School of Medicine, USA) and Stephanie Bowlin (Western University of Health Sciences, USA)
Medical Information Science Reference • © 2020 • 371pp • H/C (ISBN: 9781799830665) • US $225.00

Handbook of Research on the Efficacy of Training Programs and Systems in Medical Education
Ruth Gotian (Weill Cornell Medicine, USA) Yoon Kang (Weill Cornell Medicine, USA) and Joseph Safdieh (Weill Cornell Medicine, USA)
Medical Information Science Reference • © 2020 • 566pp • H/C (ISBN: 9781799814689) • US $365.00

Gender Equity in the Medical Profession
Maria Irene Bellini (Belfast Health and Social Care Trust, UK) and Vassilios E. Papalois (Imperial College London, UK)
Medical Information Science Reference • © 2020 • 339pp • H/C (ISBN: 9781522595991) • US $265.00

For an entire list of titles in this series, please visit:
http://www.igi-global.com/book-series/advances-medical-education-research-ethics/132365

IGI Global
PUBLISHER of TIMELY KNOWLEDGE

701 East Chocolate Avenue, Hershey, PA 17033, USA
Tel: 717-533-8845 x100 • Fax: 717-533-8661
E-Mail: cust@igi-global.com • www.igi-global.com

Table of Contents

Detailed Table of Contents

Since birth, humans absorb information from what surrounds them. Kindergartens, schools, and universities work as institutions to insert everyone in a culturally similar environment, giving equal educational opportunities to future citizens. These institutions develop human competencies for a society enabled to feed everyone, to sustain healthcare, and to protect the environment. This effort implies educational performances, whose grounds should rely on theories of learning and different modes of teaching. Pharmacy faculties, apart from teaching, reinforcing, and updating the students' knowledge on pharmaceutical sciences, guide students towards respecting different health professionals, aware of their role as educational supporters of patients and families who use pharmacies as the closest advising and health caring places. This is especially important nowadays, with the complexity of some diseases and the rising costs of healthcare. This chapter gives an overview of pharmacy teaching and learning according to the European Association of Faculties of Pharmacy.

The purpose of this chapter is to further explore how the global vision for the future of pharmacy education shared by many stakeholders and catalyzed by the launch of the workforce development goals by the International Federation of Pharmacy (FIP) was transformed into a specific cluster of academic goals. In this chapter, the expected impact of the Pharmaceutical Workforce Development Goals in academia and pharmacy education will be further explored, with a special focus on a consensual group of statements that would be become known as "The Nanjing Statements." The chapter explores how all these factors contributed to the change of the way the pharmaceutical workforce is educated, and how the challenge is currently being met.

Healthcare professionals, especially pharmacists, are constantly involved with drug information and should be able to properly select resources and keep updated on new literature and new tools to address a variety of drug information requests. The provision of accurate in-depth drug information requires the development of drug information skills through both didactic and experiential training programs. Considering the complexity of the drug information field and the expanding roles of pharmacists as information resources, this chapter will briefly introduce the main concepts of drug information and discuss the potential methods and challenges for teaching this subject while matching the variety of learning styles.

Evidence-based practice is a key element and indicator of high-quality patient care. Healthcare professionals must effectively acquire the necessary knowledge, skills, and attitudes to gather, assess, and interpret the best available evidence in order to ground their clinical decisions. Both achieving competency and delivering instruction in evidence-based practice are complex processes requiring a multimodal approach that may include traditional lectures, interactive teaching strategies, clinically-integrated teaching strategies, active learning. This chapter will provide a brief overview of the concepts of evidence-based practice, interpretation of systematic reviews and meta-analyses, grading evidence, and recommendations' strength. For each topic, teaching strategies or methods will be discussed.

implemented in a pharmacy law and ethics module. The perspectives of students collected through surveys were overall favorable. These perspectives, together with other favorable indicators, led to TBL maintenance until the current days.

Clinical research is a large umbrella, and it mainly includes the implementation of clinical studies/trials. This field is crucial to assess the value of new developments in healthcare, be it new therapeutic interventions, medical devices, or systems of care. In order to protect human rights, the implementation of clinical trials is complex and extremely costly. In this context, medicines and medical devices are strongly regulated products before and after the market authorization. So during their training, pharmacists must develop skills in the area of regulatory affairs, design and methodology of clinical trials, and other clinical studies, as well as in the management of clinical projects to be prepared for the challenges of the clinical research and market access processes. With that purpose, knowledge and skills for clinical research should be developed in association with regulatory affairs.

Professional practice is regulated by associations with regulatory powers, namely the Portuguese Pharmaceutical Society (PPS). Education is regulated by the Ministry of Education, responsible for ensuring access to quality of education for all citizens across all professional spectra. Aiming to contribute to an improved continuity between education and the career pathway, from early phases to eventual specialization, the PPS, who represents the interests of all registered pharmacists, developed a new structure entitled the Education and Practice Platform (EPP). This structure includes one representative from each institution providing education in pharmaceutical sciences and all Councils of Specialty Boards of Practice. This chapter provides an

Foreword

The Editors of this book invited me to foreword this volume and I am honored for two main reasons. Firstly, because it is a book with a very important theme, and through it, readers will find intelligible teaching practices and methods in the field of pedagogies for Pharmacy Curricula. Secondly, the authors are all very experienced academics, teaching students and pharmacists for many years and this book shows important perspectives presenting current and emerging opportunities. I should say that this is the work we have been waiting for many years, to lead both academic and professional communities to boost the utmost important debate on the quality and adequacy of education for young pharmacists, aiming the necessary alignment between education and practice, in light of predicting fitness for practice.

The pharmacists' scope of practice has been expanded worldwide, following the international trends of Health Systems Transition for more dynamic and innovative care approaches, multidisciplinary and evidenced-based, e-health driven, as well as using big data for producing real-world evidence which monitors health outcomes, bringing clinical value to patients and their careers. All this transformation, from a more static health system to an improving health care system, has to be followed by a strong focus on how future pharmaceutical workforces should be trained for taking into account the framework of competencies that are foreseen as needed for a multidisciplinary patient lead health care delivery.

While reading this book, one becomes extremely enthusiastic with all the strategic science-based thinking that the authors presented in a very elegant, clear and open-minded way. I am sure every single reading will add value enlightening the complex and fundamental debate on the future of the pharmacist profession, paving the way for new opportunities.

Finally, I would like to express my deep gratitude to all the authors for the wonderful work they have done, that will help the entire community in the mission of shaping the future of pharmacist education. *Sydney Harris* wrote that "the whole purpose of education is to turn mirrors into windows". I like to think that this book will help all of us pharmacists, pharmacy scientists and academics to see through these windows the future we need and deserve, in order to help patients worldwide becoming healthier and happier, thus fulfilling our purpose.

Ana Paula Martins
Portuguese Pharmaceutical Society, Lisbon, Portugal

Ana Paula Martins *is Professor of Pharmacoepidemiology & Pharmacovigilance and President of the Portuguese Pharmaceutical Society (Ordem dos Farmacêuticos).*

Preface

Higher education is a dynamic ecosystem that must be sensitive to social changes and technological developments. Responding to these challenges imply that course curricula for professional education and training can adapt and evolve towards pedagogical alternatives and creative teaching solutions.

As with other fast development areas, adaptive behavior is crucial to pharmaceutical education and related training. The pharmaceutical practices and their output are an unequivocal example of such developments: practice in previous decades is remarkably different from the evolving roles and additional pharmacists' expectations as healthcare service providers.

The increase in the skillset and associated educational demand, the expanding pharmaceutical professional environments, particularly the clinical and industrial areas, require all pharmaceutical educators' combined efforts to update Schools of Pharmacy curricula that deliver the best match to government and societal expectations.

INSIDE THIS BOOK

The first chapter highlights the importance of higher education pharmacy institutions and their ability to provide knowledge in pharmaceutical sciences and guide students towards acknowledging and respecting the different healthcare players. Faculty should promote students' awareness of their role as educational supporters of patients and pharmacists as a primary source of health advice and care.

The second chapter explores a global vision for pharmacy education's future within the International Federation of Pharmacy (FIP) goals and their impact on academic education and the pharmaceutical workforce, more specifically regarding the "The Nanjing Statements."

The third chapter is on teaching and learning methods for Drug Information. It discusses the pharmacist's pivotal role in providing accurate, in-depth evidence to various drug information requests. For this to occur, both students, teachers, and other healthcare professionals should understand the main concepts of this field and recognize the challenges for teaching this subject while matching the variety of learning styles. Reliable training is critical to expanding further the pharmacist's role as a drug information provider.

The fourth chapter highlights the current challenges in evidence-based practice education, including achieving competency and delivering instructions that may better integrate evidence into clinical decision-making. Thus, this chapter provides an overview of the several teaching approaches that can be effective in this field and should be considered together with other acquired knowledge, skills, and healthcare professionals' attitudes.

The fifth chapter is centered around developing the pharmaceutical and clinical roles and the more traditional pharmaceutical knowledge education. This patient-centered attitude may be accomplished by exploring emerging opportunities regarding pharmacists' interaction with patients, which are offered by increasing Health Humanities and Narrative Medicine's inclusion to the academic curricula.

The sixth chapter presents a global vision of pharmacy as a direct provider of services, from disease prevention to therapeutic monitoring, while ensuring availability and safety. Additionally, it contextualizes the importance of aligning pharmacists' education and social needs and the need to further invest in the pharmacy workforce of the future, considering the Universal Health Coverage and the FIP Sustainable Development Goal 3.

The seventh chapter introduces Team-based Learning (TBL) in a pharmacy law and ethics module as an active learning strategy built on individual advanced preparation, readiness assurance, and team application. It provides several insights that, in addition to other indicators, explain TBL's maintenance in pharmacy education until the present day.

The eighth chapter introduces clinical research and its vital aspect in assessing new healthcare developments such as therapeutic interventions, medical devices, and other care systems. It emphasizes pharmacists' need to develop training in regulatory affairs, design, and clinical trials methodology and their management.

The last chapter provides an overview of pharmacy education in Portugal, discusses the current educational systems' strengths and limitations, and details the development, contribution, and future expectations of the Education and Practice Platform (EPP). This structure includes a representative from each pharmaceutical science institution and all Councils of Specialty Boards of Practice.

CONCLUSION

The present book presents a selection of pedagogical approaches covering different, but essential, aspects of pharmaceutical education and workforce development. Systematic strategies are presented, and prospects are discussed, aiming to foster the discussion about pharmaceutical education's future within a concerted effort by national and international entities. Only with deeply integrated, multidisciplinary, technologically advanced education, grounded on ethics, and informed by social sciences, should pharmacists maintain their crucial role in healthcare.

Section 1

Pedagogical Methodologies Perspectives in Pharmacy Curricula

Chapter 1
Perspectives on Learning and Teaching Science:
Influence on Clinical Pharmacy Education

Maria José de Almeida
CFisUC, University of Coimbra, Portugal

Isabel Vitória Figueiredo
Faculty of Pharmacy, University of Coimbra, Portugal

Maria Margarida Caramona
Faculty of Pharmacy, University of Coimbra, Portugal

ABSTRACT

Since birth, humans absorb information from what surrounds them. Kindergartens, schools, and universities work as institutions to insert everyone in a culturally similar environment, giving equal educational opportunities to future citizens. These institutions develop human competencies for a society enabled to feed everyone, to sustain healthcare, and to protect the environment. This effort implies educational performances, whose grounds should rely on theories of learning and different modes of teaching. Pharmacy faculties, apart from teaching, reinforcing, and updating the students' knowledge on pharmaceutical sciences, guide students towards respecting different health professionals, aware of their role as educational supporters of patients and families who use pharmacies as the closest advising and health caring places. This is especially important nowadays, with the complexity of some diseases and the rising costs of healthcare. This chapter gives an overview of pharmacy teaching and learning according to the European Association of Faculties of Pharmacy.

DOI: 10.4018/978-1-7998-4486-0.ch001

INTRODUCTION

Learning is simultaneously an intuitive animals' born in aptitude, but also, if considered as an enterprise taken up to its utmost level, learning can be a very complex and multifaceted mental organization based on several attitudes, motivations, and different mental efforts.Since the last decades of the XIX century, psychology has tried to explain how animals learn.

The first scientific learning theories found fundaments on irrational animals' behavior, mainly developing memorization encouraged by immediate rewards. Studies on human learning started producing learning theories in the second and third decades of the XX century when Dewey, Piaget, Vygotsky, and others wrote about learning theories based on the due rational development of human minds. Pharmacists are educated to work with technological products based on applications of scientific knowledge aiming at the improvement of human health and quality of life. Hence, pharmacists must learn basic Natural and Physical sciences, together with their different pharmacological applications. To fulfill adequately their role in publics' attendance and health care, envisaging a patient-centered pharmaceutical practice, they have also to develop pedagogical knowledge and competences, including communication, planning, forecasting, and digital soft skills.

Pharmacists should acquire the right mixture of abilities to deal with the most probable social, scientific, and technological changes one envisages on health care soon. They must be open and motivated to look for lifelong learning, either provided by health institutions or created by health care professionals participating in communities of practice, where members help colleagues developing inquiries and research projects. Pharmacists must be prepared to participate in helping the development of new models of health care collaborating with teams of physicians and other health professionals.

This work reports on physical sciences general methodologies developed during physics teachers' pre-service and in-service professional education, applied to the education of pharmacists especially in what concerns the advantages of a strong Clinical Pharmacy component for quality enhancement of the society's health care systems.

BACKGROUND

How Human Beings Learn

Since birth, humans start absorbing information from what surrounds them. Babies recognize their mothers and the close family, most especially those who feed them and heal their bruises. Children very quickly understand that parents will attend them if they cry. Infants try hard to go on sleeping with their mothers, if possible, forever.

According to constructivism (Piaget, 1969), human beings absorb, and process information perceived from the environment. We hear, smell, taste, touch and see, and we have different feelings and emotions about different experiences (Damásio, 2011). Some things we like better than other ones and some others we dislike. We start growing ideas about the world where we leave on and we try to process them within our thinking schemes. One can say that almost since birth humans' start 'modeling' in their minds the world where we all exist and try to adapt our own behavior to the perceived surroundings.

Specific human being's ideas can be different from the ones of their close neighbors. For instance, among the students of any 7th-grade physics classroom, almost everybody thinks differently about what makes an arrow fly away from the bow without falling straightly down due to gravity. Everyone's ideas depend on what private situations one has already experienced and on the self-processing of these experiences within previously existing information. Hence, personal ideas about whatever we think about depending on our family, culture, and society where we live on.

Kindergartens and schools work as institutions to insert children and youths in a culturally similar environment, giving equal educational opportunities to every future citizen. National schools have the same programs to enculture every student. Today's Basic and Secondary schools educate teenagers to become the country's adults within 10 or 15 years: they are supposed to develop knowledge and understanding on different basic subjects, believed to constitute the grounds for everyone living in our dynamic society. Today's youth must develop competence to be able in the future to find ways of feeding and caring for each other, contributing, as a society, to the protection of the Earth's environment and the progress of humanity.

It is within compulsory schooling that governments can ensure the future of humankind. The new generations must acquire today the already developed knowledge, which will function as the background of the cognitive structures of the future citizens, which must be able to push away the frontiers of knowledge. Today's students must be trained to develop adequate skills and competencies to become future scientists, medical doctors, nurses, pharmacists, lawyers, teachers and all other professions supporting an organized society.

Theories of Learning

It is common knowledge that one does not learn everything exactly in the same way. One does not learn Physics as one learns History or a foreign language. One does not learn to play the piano as one learns to present and defend its own ideas. Hence, since the end of the XIX century, psychologists have developed several important theories of learning (Phillips and Soltis, 2009). Of these, three of them are especially important when one wants to consider the learning of natural and physical sciences.

Behaviorism

Based on what scientists considered the core of scientific knowledge – the ability to perform experiments repeatable by colleagues in different institutions with similar results – the first theory of learning grew during the last decades of the XIX century.

Starting from experimental results obtained by direct observation of learning progresses made by several animals - cats, dogs, monkeys, pigeons, etc.- when subjected to different stimuli, 'behaviorism' (Watson,1930) reported details of performances illustrating experiences with irrationals. It became evident that training, repeating and rewarding animals, trying to induce memorization, made them learn how to reach special objectives.

Hence, these were then considered as the main ingredients to produce animal learning. Later, in the second half of the XX century, Skinner, 1961, used developed 'behavioristic' learning theories to build a teaching machine to help children's learning in schools.

'Behaviorism' influenced schoolteachers' professional education almost up to the end of the XX century. It led to teachers acting as explainers, producing long and uninterrupted presentations of new content, asking students to answer short direct questions and to solve simple exercises by substituting values in formulas. Teachers should reward quiet students, that are orderly listening and trying to memorize what teachers say; teachers were due to ask students to write "correct" sentences on their notebooks and later to reproduce them on texts and exams. Schools should promote the existence of "Honor boards" with lists of students obtaining very high marks in direct examinations.

Constructivism and Cognitivism

These two theories developed along the XX century and are especially devoted to human beings learning. According to them, human beings construct ('constructivism', Piaget, 1969) their own knowledge since early childhood, observing and actively processing ('cognitivism', Dewey, 1969 and Ausubel, 1963) the information obtained from their own environment, trying to integrate new knowledge into what they knew beforehand. Parents' and teachers' influences, and group experiences, can be very important to help and correctly guide this processing ('social constructivism', Vygotsky, 1978).

One continuously builds its own ideas within mental models (Greca and Moreira, 2000), consciously accommodating new knowledge into what one previously knows. Group work helps to share previous knowledge and to be aware of peers and owns developing metacognition, giving stronger support to learning in schools. This can happen through talking to each other, dialoguing, discussing, offering arguments, questioning and contacting with different ways of understanding. Different learners, eventually with different cultures and backgrounds, need different modes of teaching and coaching to be able to reach the highest potential of their own mental models' development.

Hence: 1) teaching methodologies have to be specifically student-centered and not only designed and delivered as a "one size fits all"; and 2) new information has to be processed by motivated students, aware of the need for their active participation in the teaching/learning processes. One very important role of teachers is to be able to motivate students to the point of getting them deeply involved in the development of their own learning.

By the end of the XX century, neurophysiological studies' advances gave a strong positive impact on 'constructivism' and 'cognitivism' as being the basic learning theories behind the meaningful development of people's mental models. Once scientific knowledge and scientific developments rely on scientific models developed by human minds over the centuries, the importance of these two learning theories for anyone enrolled in natural and physical sciences studies is far too evident.

Most recently, Damásio (2011), has outlined the importance of feelings and emotions on human beings' attitudes and motivations, hence on the development of mentally active enterprises.

MODES OF TEACHING

Having a fair idea of how one learns is pertinent to elaborate on the efficacy of possible modes of teaching. Skinner (2010), presents only four different teaching methodologies, which he describes deeply, pointing towards the distinct roles teachers and learners should keep whenever developing any of these teaching modes in a classroom. The author recommends that most of the time teachers should use a sequence of these different ways of teaching, in order to reach every student and to be able to produce effective learning for everyone.

The next few lines give the characteristics and real-life common examples of the use of different modes of teaching. As one can see, the proposed teaching modes are not too much different from what efficient professors generally develop within their university teaching.

Direct Teaching

It is the most common way of teaching anything to anyone, and it is the teaching mode used when the teacher talks to the whole class about some new subject, explaining new concepts, or introducing scientific laws. When we give a straight answer, producing information to someone who asks a straight question, or when we give references recognized by the learner and produce some examples of similar situations, we are practicing 'direct teaching'. It generally is the first teaching mode one uses to help any learner to try to process correctly some new information, an intermediate step very important for the future adequate use of the learners' processed new knowledge.

Thinking in terms of university teaching, one can consider Theoretical Classes as using mainly 'direct teaching'. However, for the students' efficient learning of the newly acquired knowledge, teachers must be aware of the need to keep students active, paying attention and trying to process learning at any moment. Otherwise, if attending only as passive listeners, the students will not profit very much from these classes.

Teaching Through Dialog and Discussion

It is a fundamental way of processing newly obtained knowledge when students try to explain what they understand based on previously learned content. It happens whenever someone expresses their own thoughts by words, orally or writing, when solving a problem "in loud voice", or when explaining some experimentally obtained results in terms of deep processing of recently learned concepts.

Eventually, within groups, learners use their own words to explain what they have previously understood or what they envisage as expectable from an experiment; by dialoguing and by producing arguments, learners share understanding among each other or with the teacher, exchanging, reinforcing or reformulating own ideas.

At the university, this generally happens in Practical or Theoretic-Practical classes. Again, teachers must be careful in promoting the active participation of students and the necessary collaboration of every student in group work. Asking the students to discuss some examples and to explain their mental models' evolution, teachers should notice eventual misconceptions and find ways to orient the learners towards the correct deepest level of understanding of the focused concepts.

Teaching by Action and Experience

This mode of teaching overlaps with the previous one when teachers design experiences and help learners to collect and process experimental results, interpreted according to previously obtained knowledge. This learning model also applies to learners immersed within a labor place, where future workers learn how to perform professional functions, observing and participating within a community of practice (for instance, pharmacy stages in hospitals or teachers stages in schools).

Learning occurs by careful observation, asking questions, enrolling in discussions and imitation of good professionals during their professional work. This methodology also applies when one learns how to swim, cycle, or cook a meal. After knowing the main rules eventually explained by a 'direct method', most of the learning completes by watching and trying to do it. Furthermore, most university professional degrees use this teaching model when they contain a compulsory final stage within working places, before completion.

Teaching by Inquiry

This is a mode of teaching with two main learning proposes:

1. Learners have to use previous knowledge to solve a real-life holistic scientific or professional problem, and doing so, they process deeper previous meaningfully learned science.
2. The inquiry-developed actions must follow the rules of scientific and professional research: hence, students learn, in practice, how science and professional behaviors develop, something the society expects them to continue.

In the 'inquiry', individuals or group members start by presenting and discussing hypotheses to solve an existing problem and try to agree on an experimental design believed to be a way to allow the decision about the problem's solutions. Students must execute the experiments, using appropriate instruments for data collection. They interpret the obtained results, reflecting on their meaning and developed experimental work. Finally, the individual or the group must present their work and conclusions, submitting all the process to the teacher and peers' acknowledgment and discussion.

There are different levels of 'inquiry', according to the students' learning levels and respecting the amount of previously acquired knowledge: sometimes teachers produce some guidelines to orient the learners, or give some previous scaffolding, or let the students work on their own. On the most independent inquiries, learners must design themselves in their own scientific ways and to look for the necessary instruments to reach the defined objectives.

At the university, natural and physical science students start using guided 'inquiry' methods on their experimental projects and monographs included in first university degrees. One can say that Master students go on developing ever-independent scientific and professional 'inquiries' and, finally, that Ph.D. students work within the professional and scientific research levels.

GENERAL CONCERNS OF PHARMACISTS' EDUCATION

Apart from the fundamentals of scientific knowledge on physics and chemistry, pharmacists must learn pharmaceuticals, pharmacology, pharmacodynamics, pharmacotherapy, pharmacoepidemiology, and others adequate to help them to attend to their pharmacy users' needs.

They must also dominate social skills based on empathy, motivation and respect enabling them to reach people of different levels of education and to demonstrate attention towards their doubts and specific problems. In order to be efficient, all this knowledge and competences acquisition imply correctly designed sequences of teaching methods, organized according to the learning theories, as well as a due assessment of students' understanding (Strang and Baia, 2016).

Pharmacists must be educated and trained to give pharmaceutical help to persons of very different ages and educational levels. For some users, a simple explanation is enough, but others may also need personal comfort and deep empathy. Pharmacists must be able to explain eventual compulsory rules, which must be understandable by everyone who listens to them. They must be aware that sometimes they must encourage and motivate pharmacy users to follow difficult protocols they cannot understand deeply.

THE CONTENT APPROACH OF PHARMACY LEARNING

Nowadays, in many countries all around the world following the recent reports of the International Pharmacists Federation (FIP) and of the World Health Organization (WHO) a pharmacist is a health professional with responsibilities in efficient, safe and economical use of medicines by individuals and by the society.

It is relevant in this context to consider the pharmaceutical profession as a whole and to understand the main area of pharmacists' activities focused on the medicines. Medicine is a drug, or a single chemical substance, a natural product or a biotechnological preparation used to prevent or to treat diseases, or to alter a physiological function.

Medicines are single drugs, or a mixture of drugs combined with other substances, prepared on a pharmaceutical formulation, in a variety of forms, for a route of administration.

These forms include tablets, capsules, solutions, creams, ointments, suppositories, injectable, modified released products, or other adequate forms used in new presentations. After administration, every drug is locally absorbed into the blood and distributed throughout the body.

From there begins the pharmacological process where the ADME (absorption, distribution, metabolism and excretion) of the active substance have specific locals to act and a normally expected therapeutic effect.

At the same time or subsequently, the active compounds suffer a metabolic process to obtain both the pharmacological results and the expected therapeutic outcomes.

Finally, either altered or not in their chemical or biotechnological characteristics, they are excreted from the body.

Drugs interact with tissues and organs altering their function and these effects are not always desirable. Sometimes the side effects or the collateral responses can be a risk to the patient or cause inefficacy of the treatment.

DISEASES AND WELLBEING

The disease is a phenomenon closely linked with human life and every human being has the duty and right to prevent or treat it. Since the 1960s the WHO considers health as *a complete state of physical, mental and social well-being, and not just the absence of disease.*

Today's societies accept medicines (or drugs) as primer commodities and necessary goods with technically advanced therapeutic formulations, under severe and complex regulations even on economic grounds.

Throughout their life cycle, medicines are subject to technical and legal compliance with strong demands of Quality, Effectiveness and Safety standards, which the regulatory authorities of each country verify and reinforce.

Research for new drugs, development and manufacturing processes, authority permissions and marketing rules, distribution channels, prescribing, dispensing, surveillance after authorization and pharmacovigilance are subjected to numerous legislative and technical standards.

COMMUNITY AND HOSPITAL PHARMACISTS

Pharmacists within the community and hospitals are medication-use experts. We all live through rapid changes in health care strategies for the profession. The movements to orient patients and develop pharmaceutical care must grow in the community, in the hospital, in patients at home, and with those living in nursing homes.

Pharmaceutical education must acknowledge the importance of multiple medication problems, preparing services to monitor the follow-up of outpatients under treatment, including potentially the detection of harm of misused medication and preventing hospital admission or readmission.

The prescription needs to be rational in the medications use when it is necessary to decide or to choose within a clinical situation which medicines to apply. Health systems must rationalize the use of health technologies and medicines because the economic systems that support medical services are struggling in every country with the budgetary balance requirements for each one.

In the applicability of the principles of rationality for the prescription of medicines and their use in a hospital or outpatient setting, health professionals should participate in the uncompromising defense of these principles. They benefit the patients, the citizens, and society.

LEARNING AND MISSION OF PHARMACISTS

According to Manasse (1990), the mission of a pharmacist is to serve society as the professional responsible for the appropriate use of medication, medical devices and support services to achieve optimal therapeutic outcomes. The cited author attributes to the pharmacist the responsibility to ensure that the medication regime adapts to the individual patient, based on the correct diagnosis accepted by the clinical parameters and on the pharmacological knowledge about the medicines selected for the treatment.

A wide variety of medications, new products, and new services are available today in the health system. With the specific orientation of the health professional team, we can attribute to the pharmacists the big role of being the informers about medicines and medical devices.

One of the main objectives of the European Society of Clinical Pharmacy, ESCP, founded in 1979, was to stimulate and improve the education of pharmacists in the orientation of the clinical pharmacy. Since then, according to this society, a clinical pharmacist is *a health care provider promoting the effective, safe and economic use of drugs by individuals and by society.*

The educational objectives for clinical pharmacists are not only valuable for hospital pharmacists but also community pharmacists because, although the patient-oriented pharmacy activities start in hospitals, the work to rationalize the use of medicines pertains also to the ambulatory and the primary care.

According to an Education Document by Bonal (1988), edited by ESCP, the institutional objectives for the education of a clinical pharmacist are:

1. Ensure that each patient receives appropriate drug therapy according to his individual needs.
2. Contribute to the determination of the benefits/risk of drug therapy for each patient, as well as for the community.

3. Interact responsibly with all persons involved in the provision of health care.
4. Educate patients and health care professionals to promote safe, effective and appropriate drug use.
5. Promote the cost/effective use of drugs.
6. Perform research to improve drug therapy.
7. Obtain information and learn how to improve practice.
8. Evaluate the individual performances, identify and correct any deficiencies, and be updated with this knowledge.

Concerning practice improvement, both in education and research, we must consider that the education and training of the professionals allied to a high multidisciplinary team dialogue are relevant to the updated preparation of the clinical pharmacist.

Educating pharmacists to adopt a clinical approach requires knowledge, skills, and attitudes in addition to their pharmaceutical sciences. This additional expertise should enable pharmacists to apply their acquired knowledge to improve the care of patients.

Another document from ESCP, 1988, contains in the introduction the following citation, useful to the comprehension of the above-mentioned requirements, that *all pharmacists need to develop some of the knowledge, skills, and attitudes necessary for a clinical pharmacy approach but the extent and degree of specialization in these developments will vary depending on the degree of direct clinical involvement of the Hospital Pharmacist with the patient and prescriber.*

The WHO report published in 1994 recognizes that the clinical involvement of the community pharmacists is potentially as great as that of the hospital pharmacists.

Much of said knowledge and attitudes, together with some skills, can start through 'direct teaching' or using 'discussions and dialogues' and training in the classrooms at the undergraduate level. However, the full development of good clinical practices requires suitable training in the practice environment, with characteristics of 'teaching by action and experience', where learners can learn from each other and the contact with good professionals.

REQUIREMENTS TO BE A COMPETENT PROFESSIONAL

What knowledge, contents and skills should be the 'educational luggage' of a competent pharmacist? On a concise answer, one must say:

1. Pharmaceutical knowledge – in pharmaceutical chemistry, pharmaceutics, pharmacology, therapeutics and other subjects enabling a deep understanding

of the main areas of the profession. This is a consequence of believing that the medicines need to be correctly prepared and correctly used. It is a type of knowledge obtainable and duly applied to real situations through direct teaching, teaching by dialog and discussion, and teaching by action and experience.

2. Clinical knowledge – to be aware of the most common diseases of the body systems. To establish the connection between the clinical situation and the disease factors. To be able to grow a reasonable understanding of the physician's desires and patient needs. To express the ability to interview patients in order to obtain a short medical history before counter dispensing or medicines history prior to hospital admission. To be able to effectively educate patients in the use of prescribed and over the counter medicines. This knowledge develops better and deeper through 'inquiry' (group work on practical cases problem solving) and 'teaching by action and experience' (stages within working places).
3. Social and behavioral awareness – to consider the patient as a psycho and social entity at the center of a process who needs information about their medicines and the effects of them. In addition, pharmacists should respect the relations with physicians, nurses and other health professionals, important for the benefice of the patient. Again, this knowledge and competences should complement and further develop within working places.
4. Public Health organization with management of economic factors influencing illness, health and medicines use. Pharmacists must consider the real quality of life of the patients and the costs of healthcare. This type of learning can better develop through writing and discussing monographs, the organization of role-playing sessions, or the development of 'inquiry projects'.

Apart from the general approach we have presented up to now, we cannot forget the social importance of the biomedical tests used to diagnose and monitor disease and responses to medical therapy. In addition, one should focus the clinical applications of pharmacokinetics and biopharmaceutics on patient care or the clinical application of the pharmaceuticals drug delivery systems, or biostatistics and epidemiology, or clinical nutrition particularly by the parenteral route, and policies for monitoring and controlling infections. These contents must integrate the different curricular disciplines of the Pharmacy courses.

RESEARCH IN PRACTICE – CHALLENGES AND OPPORTUNITIES

To be able to educate pharmacists up to the high standards above defined, one needs strong and organized cooperation between schools of pharmacy, hospitals, other health research institutions and the professionals. Together they constitute the main forces to change and greatly improve the pharmacy practice. Furthermore, the organization of continuing professional education after the master's degree completion is fundamental, allowing the progress of pharmacists on ever implementing their preservice obtained knowledge. In 2014, the FIP congress organized one main session on "Science-based pharmacy towards better medicines and patients care" and on "Access to medicines and pharmacists today, better outcomes tomorrow".

Nowadays with highly potent and complex pharmaceutical agents available for the treatment of diseases, the need for information about medicines for patients, physicians and health professionals has greatly increased. Additionally, the related research on the morbidity and mortality due to the use of medicines and the rising costs associated with new promising medicines and associated treatments constitute substantive knowledge fundamental for the pharmacists.

The adequate use of medicines significantly increases the control of health problems, correcting the poor outcomes of badly used pharmacotherapies through ineffective and unsafe treatments and this responsibly pertains to the pharmacists. In the WHO Assembly in Tokyo (1993), the members called attention to the need for support for the development of a patient-centered practice focused on Pharmaceutical Care. The Assembly has recognized and strengthened this concept. In 1994, the WHO published the report "The Role of the Pharmacist in Health Care System".

In 1999, a medical assembly from the World Medical Association produced a statement on the working relationship between physicians and pharmacists in medical therapy, recognizing the important roles of pharmacists.

From it, we can transcribe the five main points:

1. To provide information to patients, which may include the name of the medicines, its purpose, potential interactions and side effects as well as correct usage and storage.
2. To review prescription orders to identify interactions, allergic reactions, contraindications and therapeutic duplications.
3. On the patient's request, to discuss medicine-related problems and concerns about the prescribed medicines.
4. To report to health authorities received information about adverse reactions of medicines, whenever appropriate.
5. To maintain a high level of knowledge about medicinal therapy through continuing professional development.

All these procedures rely on a patient-oriented service, within a perspective of pharmaceutical care services. One should monitor the process of medicines use from a preventive perspective: identifying the eventual risks in the treatment; acting within the dispensing in the analysis of the morbidity indicators and the medication review; monitoring the outcomes from a reactive attitude, identifying the negative ones by pharmacotherapy follow-up and disease management.

The position paper of EAFP 2018 describes the competencies for pharmaceutical care, also focused on the ESCP 1993 document. One should teach contents on the specific knowledge about medicines from the user perspective oriented to the patients understanding their diseases to ensure the correct rational and economic use of drugs and to obtain better compliance. Concerning skills, the referred documents purpose an emphatic and strong practical educational component on communication skills.

Another educational practical component refers to learning how to translate scientific perspectives into daily practical outcomes; furthermore, pharmacists should be able to act as team players within interdisciplinary health teams.

In every learning phase, the students' attitudes must be inquisitive, objective, diligent, cooperative and empathic. Students should also be educated to accept the ethical professional orientations and deontological principles of pharmacists and to be open and actively willing to participate in lifelong learning and innovative and digital networking learning.

Pharmacists need to know how to use updated information to support the scientific-based decisions and individual health critical analysis; to develop ethical behavior and capacities to contribute to health teamwork; and leadership. Within the technical competence and knowledge, solid training in pharmaceutical sciences is relevant mainly in pathophysiology, pharmacology, and pharmacotherapy. The ability to systematize and register the actions and consequences in each case and problem solved is also fundamental.

Summarizing: communication skills, scientific knowledge and update information about medicines are the bases to implement health promotion and disease prevention. To point out and conclude, when pharmacists and physicians work together, recognizing their own roles to ensure the safe and appropriate use of medicines, one is prepared to achieve the best health outcomes for the patients.

PHARMACISTS IN THE HEALTH SYSTEM

One can consider that the main responsibility of the pharmacist is both to the patient´s well-being and the Health System. The involvement of the pharmacist in the evaluation of clinical results produced by the medicines can contribute to the reduction of morbidity and mortality associated with them, assisting patients to obtain the maximum benefit from the medications. Pharmacists must have general and specific knowledge enabling them to watch the patient both in yield and following the pharmacotherapy, interacting with the patient and other professionals, aiming at improving the patients´ quality of life and the stable accountability of the Health System.

The changes in health policies with a focus on primary care allow the pharmacist to play a role in pharmaceutical care services in the regional Health Department of Primary Care. Some European countries have promoted the integration of pharmacists in the development of a National Formulary of Medicines, used in the national hospitals and in Ambulatory Health Sections.

There they provide expert pharmaceutical advice to inform the cost-effective delivery of expensive new therapy and lifestyle drugs. The Formulary guidelines have numerous associated benefits such as cost-effective integrations of primary and secondary prescriptions, increased knowledge on new therapies, and support provided for general practitioners and community pharmacists sharing responsibilities for monitoring the therapies.

Community pharmacists are assuming the role of medication advisers and assist patients in the management of their medication. Further, the increased deregulation of drugs available for over the counter sale and the access to the computerized patient medication records existing in hospitals enabled pharmacists to advise and treat a wider range of patients' minor symptoms.

Science background in Pharmacy education enables pharmacists to approach all fields of pharmacotherapy, the classical and the emerging ones, such as the advanced therapies, the efficacy/safety assessment through the adaptive pathways approach, and the effectiveness evaluation through Big data analysis (mainly due to the large numbers of individuals and the depth of data on each individual).

According to Morais and Caramona (2019), the efforts to improve timely access for patients to new medicines in European Medicines Agency support the adaptive pathways approach. This is a scientific concept for medicine development and data generation, allowing for early and real patient access to medicine.

Big data provides information and knowledge allowing new insights, revealing hidden and increased efficiencies. These tools and data will not replace the randomized clinical trials but will improve clinical trials and complement data, supporting the correct decisions on evidence for the medicines use.

The pharmacists' education should emphasize the knowledge, the skills and the competences (not forgetting empathy, assertiveness, and self-confidence) in order to achieve recognition in the society for their role as available, knowledgeable and caring professionals, available for the patients and their caretakers.

CONCLUSION

After the approach of the perspectives of teaching Physical Sciences and the influence of these on the Clinical Pharmacy Education, we decided to present, as a conclusion, some of the patterns where pharmacists develop and apply their knowledge and developed competences on professional research in cooperation with other health professionals.

In general, one uses questionnaires to assess adherence to the therapeutic regimen, and some of these questionnaires are validated via self-administration. Sometimes, the inadequate health literacy of the elderly pushes researchers to use interviews as a method of questionnaire administration.

Cabral et al. (2017), report on the influence of the mode of administration of questionnaires, comparing the results obtained with interviewer-administered with the self-administered ones. The authors conclude that the interview administration method induced bias that led to a higher percentage of the answer "never" and a subsequent overestimated adherence levels that allowed them to conclude that self-report administration should be preferred when applying adherence questionnaires.

Figueiredo et al. (2018), report on a teaching experiment at the University of Coimbra. As defined above, the students in the Faculties of Pharmacy should be oriented and learn about the responsibility not only to dispense medicines but also to assist patients in obtaining maximum benefit from their medication when interacting with health professionals for improving their quality of life.

The Faculty of Pharmacy in Coimbra University practices these commitments, orienting teaching topics and student learning methods to these final aims. With this purpose, the Faculty of Pharmacy in Coimbra University appraises the degrees' final course supported by research-based on real practice, materialized as a written thesis, presented and discussed with a School Jury.

The Jury selected five student's works developed in community pharmacy and obtaining high final marks, with the following subjects:

1. Follow-up of diabetic patients.
2. Cardiovascular risk evaluation.
3. Medication review on elderly patients.
4. Information on the interaction with Anti-Inflammatory Non-Steroid medicines.
5. Patient's compliance with antihypertensive treatment.

The patient-centered pharmaceutical care service is a formative requirement and the need in education is increasingly justified by the useful and practical experience in the way of clinical pharmacy and pharmaceutical care.

It is also relevant to mention the work performed and the practical experience shared by eight European countries for the benefit of elderly patients. The consortium SYMPATHY (Stimulating Innovation Management of Polypharmacy and Adherence in the Elderly) aims at exploring how health care management programs should develop to improve medication safety and prevent patient harm by addressing the appropriate use of multiple medications (polypharmacy).

The fundamental of these programs is the principle that providers work in partnership with the patients to enable shared decision-making regarding medication, which improves patient adherence and medicines related outcomes. From the Sympathy Project, it is possible to refer to three main approaches: Quality, Economic and Political. QUALITY means the management of polypharmacy, as an essential element of patient safety in an integrated care setting making a significant contribution to well-being. ECONOMIC refers to the prevention of harm due to medicines and can reduce demands on the healthcare system, reducing threats to the sustainability of health services. POLITICAL where the demography changes are driving up public awareness of polypharmacy issues, demanding a response from politicians and polypharmacy.

The executive summary of the project points up to six key recommendations to deliver better patients' outcomes:

Recommendation 1: Use a systems approach that has multidisciplinary clinical and policy leadership
Recommendation 2: Nurture a culture that encourages and prioritize the safety and quality of prescribing
Recommendation 3: Ensure that patients are integral to the decisions made about their medicines and are empowered and supported to do so
Recommendation 4: Use data to drive change
Recommendation 5: Adopt an evidence-based approach with a bias towards action
Recommendation 6: Utilize, develop and share tools to support the implementation

This part of the text supports the 2017 document "Polypharmacy Management by 2030: a patient safety challenge" of the SYMPATHY consortium.

As a final comment, we must say that community pharmacists are the health professionals most accessible to the public and are the cornerstones of primary health care; in the WHO, 2019, report we have the good pharmacy practice rules pointing towards the possible key players involved in the legal and regulatory framework and outlines of their missions and functions.

REFERENCES

Ausubel, D. (1963). *The psychology of meaningful verbal learning*. University Press.

Bonal, J. (1988). *The Clinical Pharmacist: Education Document*. European Society of Clinical Pharmacy.

Cabral, A., Moura-Ramos, M., Castel-Branco, M., Caramona, M., Fernandez-Llimós, F., & Figueiredo, I. V. (2017). Influence of the mode of administration on the results of medication adherence questionnaires. *Journal of Evaluation in Clinical Practice*, *23*(6), 1–6. doi:10.1111/jep.12773 PMID:28714551

Damásio, A. (2011). *O erro de Descartes. Emoção, razão e cérebro humano*. Temas e Debates – Círculo de Leitores.

Dewey, J. (1969). *The child and the curriculum and The school and Society joint edition*. University of Chicago Press, Phoenix Books.

EAFP. (2018). *Four Pillars for Relevant Pharmacy Education*. Position paper of the European Association of Faculties of Pharmacy 2018 Annual Conference, Parma, Italy.

ESCP. (1988). *Clinical Pharmacy Education and Training for Pharmacists in the European Economic Community*. European Society of Clinical Pharmacy.

ESCP. (1993). *The future of Clinical Pharmacy in Europe: A strategy for the Society* (J. Bonal, M. Burden, & J. P. Delporte, Eds.). European Society of Clinical Pharmacy.

Figueiredo, I. V., Castel-Branco, M., Fernandez-Llimós, F., & Caramona, M. (2018). Teaching topics in pharmaceutical care as a way to develop useful and practical research in community pharmacy. *Pharmacy Education: Towards Pharmaceutical Sciences*. Annual Conference of European Association of Faculties of Pharmacy. Parma, Italy.

FIP. (2014). *Access to medicines and pharmacists today, better outcomes tomorrow*. 74th World Congress of Pharmacy and Pharmaceutical Sciences. Bangkok, Thailand.

Greca, I. M., & Moreira, M. A. (2000). Mental models, conceptual models and modeling. *International Journal of Science Education*, *22*(1), 1–11. doi:10.1080/095006900289976

Manasse, H. (1990). A philosophy of education in the next millennium. *Conference on Lifelong Learning in Pharmacy*, Copenhagen, Denmark.

Morais, J. G., & Caramona, M. M. (2019). Creative Education: towards competences in a patient pharmacy education. *25th Annual conference of EAFP*. Closing session conference, Krakow, Poland.

Phillips, D. C., & Soltis, J. F. (2009). *Perspectives on Learning*. Teachers College Press, Columbia University.

Piaget, J. (1969). *Psychology of Intelligence*. Littlefield, Adams.

Skinner, B. F. (1961). Teaching Machines. In Cumulative Record. New York: Appleton-Century-Crofts. doi:10.1037/11324-011

Skinner, D. (2010). *Effective Teaching and Learning in Practice*. Continuum International Publishing Group.

Strang, A. F., & Baia, P. (2016). An investigation of teaching and learning in Pharmacy Education. *American Journal of Pharmaceutical Education*, *80*(4), 59. doi:10.5688/ajpe80459 PMID:27293226

SYMPATHY Consortium. (2017). *Polypharmacy Management by 2030: a patient safety challenge*. SYMPATHY Consortium.

Vygotsky, L. S. (1978). *Mind in Society*. Harvard University Press.

Watson, J. B. (1930). *Behaviorism*. W. W. Norton.

WHO. (1994). *The Role of the Pharmacist in the Health Care System*. Report based on a WHO meeting, Tokyo, Japan. (WHO/PHARM/94.569)

WHO. (2019). The legal and regulatory framework for community pharmacies in the WHO European Region. Copenhagen: World Health Organization, Regional Office for Europe. License: CC BY-NC-SA 3.0 IGO.

World Medical Association. (1999). Statement on the Working Relationship between Physicians and Pharmacists in Medicinal Therapy. 51st World Medical Assembly, Tel Aviv, Israel.

Chapter 2
Adapting Education to the Needs of Pharmacists and Pharmaceutical Scientists

Bruno Sepodes
Faculty of Pharmacy, University of Lisbon, Portugal

João Pedro Rocha
Faculty of Pharmacy, University of Lisbon, Portugal

Maria-Eduardo Figueira
Faculty of Pharmacy, University of Lisbon, Portugal

ABSTRACT

The purpose of this chapter is to further explore how the global vision for the future of pharmacy education shared by many stakeholders and catalyzed by the launch of the workforce development goals by the International Federation of Pharmacy (FIP) was transformed into a specific cluster of academic goals. In this chapter, the expected impact of the Pharmaceutical Workforce Development Goals in academia and pharmacy education will be further explored, with a special focus on a consensual group of statements that would be become known as "The Nanjing Statements." The chapter explores how all these factors contributed to the change of the way the pharmaceutical workforce is educated, and how the challenge is currently being met.

DOI: 10.4018/978-1-7998-4486-0.ch002

INTRODUCTION

The Global Vision for the Future of Pharmacy Education

Today it is widely accepted that people are living longer lives due to medical progress and integration of scientific knowledge and research. Many decades of innovation and investment have led to important breakthroughs in the management of patients around the world. Several global factors are contributing to the paradigm shift in the way education in health sciences, particularly in pharmacy, is faced these days.

It is undeniable that although the world population is growing, as well as the economy and commercial trade, social and economic disparities persist, and this leads to the known prevalence of poverty in some cities, regions, countries, and even entire continents.

This results in significant differences in the way health is distributed among a certain population and populations. In part, it explains why such variation exists between nations in terms of the burden of disease. Although the epidemiological transition is occurring in many countries, the burden of disease associated with communicable diseases remains an issue in many countries despite the progress made in science.

On the other hand, in the case of developed countries, mortality and morbidity are mainly related to non-communicable diseases. Additionally, how health systems are organized in each country or region varies considerably and this creates barriers associated with the accessibility and cost of health technologies and care.

The world is facing increasing globalization of healthcare, which is becoming more focused on the patient and patient's needs. The same happened to Pharmacy that is moving from a 'product-centric' approach to a 'patient-centric' focus, at least in the developed countries.

Healthcare workers are at the center of healthcare provided to populations and their training and competencies need to provide reassurance that the best care is being delivered to patients. This vision is global and embraces not only pharmacy education but also education across other areas such as medicine and nursing, to name just a few.

In its vision to 2020, the International Federation of Pharmacy (FIP) identified some pharmacy professional factors as key factors to consider when deciding upon future strategies and resulting actions to bring better healthcare to populations. They speculated that the number of trained and competent pharmacists may be either unavailable or inadequately distributed to meet population needs (FIP, 2008).

This is considered to result from different education and training processes of pharmacists and pharmaceutical scientists around the world and this highlighted the need to scrutinize these processes and find ways of improving them through both experience and research evidence (FIP, 2008).

Pharmacists are part of the broad healthcare professionals team involved in the promotion of health, prevention, and management of disease in patients. The modern pharmacist is directly providing patient care, and this is the result of an evolution from being solely concerned with primary prevention of disease to being actively involved in therapeutic monitoring (FIP, 2008).

If pharmacists are to continually contribute to the health system and to be able to actively contribute as a key player in these expected roles, an advancement is needed in the way pharmacists and pharmaceutical scientists are educated worldwide.

There is no workforce without education. Pharmacy education needs a consistent reforming spirit in order to meet the continuing challenge of training up to date professionals. It's therefore fundamental that the international community agrees on the way forward to educate competent professionals.

It is, therefore, mandatory to invest in the pharmaceutical workforce,[1] thriving to ensure access to quality essential health services, and safe and effective medicines and vaccines (FIP, 2019). This is crucial towards achieving universal health coverage by 2030 as outlined in the United Nations Sustainable Development Goals (SDGs) (United Nations, 2019). Goal 3 of the UN's SDGs is to *ensure healthy lives and promote well-being for all at all ages*, which includes "*providing access to safe, effective, quality and affordable essential medicines and vaccines for all. By providing direct access to valuable medicine expertise, the pharmaceutical workforce plays a key role in improving health outcomes through the responsible use of medicines and optimizing effective choice and use* (United Nations, 2019).

The FIP Workforce Transformation Program (WTP) is a global program that supports FIP's member organizations and stakeholders as leaders in advancing the national pharmaceutical workforces.

The program is designed to *strategically support countries in developing needs-based, national workforce development strategies, workforce planning and actions. The WTP vision is for every country to have a needs-based, national strategy and action plan for pharmaceutical workforce development* (FIP, 2019). Thus, in order to ensure the success of these global pharmaceutical programs, a joint plan on how to address global pharmacy education is crucial.

In 2013, FIP published a very comprehensive report aimed at understanding pharmacy education around the world, compiling the results from 109 participating countries (Law, Bader, Uzman, Williams, & Bates, 2019). From this report, it becomes very clear that the way we are educating pharmacists is not uniform, and there are relevant changes in both capacity and infrastructures (Law et al., 2019).

Additionally, FIP's conceptual framework of 'needs-based education' which stipulates that education and workforce development of pharmacy in any country should be directly linked to its health needs and services, is reinforced by this report (Law et al., 2019).

The FIP Centennial Declaration in 2012 stated that *Pharmacists and pharmaceutical scientists accept responsibility and accountability for improving global health and patient health outcomes by closing gaps in the development, distribution and responsible use of medicines.* (FIP, 2016a). Nevertheless, action was needed to tackle the worldwide variability existing in terms of how pharmaceutical scientists, pharmacists, and pharmacy support staff are educated and trained (FIP, 2016a).

Conscious of these needs, FIP developed a global conference to serve as a dialogue platform between universities and professional organizations so that the international community agrees on a multilevel intervention strategy in order to have a competent workforce continuously trained from a pre-graduate level to a post-graduate level. For the sake of clarity, it is important to understand what the pharmaceutical workforce is for FIP.

Across the documents published by FIP, the pharmaceutical workforce is defined as *the whole of the pharmacy-related workforce (e.g. registered pharmacist practitioners, pharmaceutical scientists, pharmacy technicians and other pharmacy support workforce cadres, pre-service students/trainees) working in a diversity of settings (e.g. community, hospital, research and development, industry, military, regulatory, academia and other sectors) with a diversity of scope of practice* (FIP, 2016b).

The global conference on pharmacy and Pharmaceutical sciences education took place in Nanjing (China) in the year 2016 and aimed to establish the milestones for impactful global development for pharmacy and pharmaceutical sciences education (FIP, 2016b). In this chapter, we will first investigate the Academic Cluster of the Workforce Development Goals and how these objectives are further reflected in the Nanjing Statements and hopefully transferred into the educational foundations of pharmacists worldwide.

BACKGROUND

Impact of the 'Pharmaceutical Workforce Development Goals' in Academia and Pharmacy Education

As a result of the efforts developed by FIP and member organizations and receiving strong inspiration from the format and content of the sustainable development goals presented by the UN for 2030 (United Nations, 2019), "pharmaceutical workforce development goals" were developed as guidance for plan actions to be developed at an international action plan to educate a stronger and committed workforce.

FIP proposed thirteen workforce development goals (WDGs) that have been grouped into three different groups (FIP, 2016b). The first group relates to 'Academy', and provides guidance for schools, universities and education providers. The second group relates to 'Professional Development' and is focused on the pharmaceutical workforce (as previously defined). Lastly, a third group relates to 'Systems' and focuses in general on policy development, governmental strategies and planning, and monitoring systems. All these levels (or groups) are considered of equal importance and all contribute to the overall goals.

The Academic Cluster

Here we will specifically focus on the Academic related cluster. Within the WDG, the academic cluster focus on all institutions connected to the education of pharmacists or, as FIP originally targeted, the pharmaceutical workforce. These institutions include schools, universities, and other education providers.

This group includes 3 workforce development goals, namely academic capacity, foundation training early career development and quality assurance.

Academic Capacity

The objective of this WDG is the *engagement with pharmaceutical higher education development policies and ready access to leaders in pharmaceutical science and clinical practice in order to support supply-side workforce development agendas* (FIP, 2016b), and these should be pursued by all those committed to the advancement of pharmacy and pharmaceutical sciences.

The rationale for investing in this development goal is thoroughly described by FIP in a public reflection paper (FIP, 2016b):

- To *increase the capacity by developing initial education and training programs that are fit for purpose, according to national health resource needs (clinical practice, pharmaceutical science areas and stakeholders across all cadres)* (FIP, 2016b).
- To *invest in the development of new and innovative ways to attract young pharmacists into all areas of pharmaceutical practice and science. This includes encouraging young pharmacists to consider careers in clinical academia, as preceptors/trainers, in industrial pharmacy, regulatory sciences, nuclear and veterinary pharmacy, among others)* (FIP, 2016b).

- The *capacity building should include the ability to meet minimum national standards of facilities, educators and student support in order to ensure access to quality education for all students* (FIP, 2016b).
- To *enhance interprofessional education and collaboration with key stakeholders, including governments, national and international pharmacy/ pharmaceutical organizations and patient advocacy groups to achieve sustainable solutions for capacity development* (FIP, 2016b).
- *The clinical academic educator workforce needs more attention to training, career development and capacity building, which must, importantly, include research capacity enhancement* (FIP, 2016b).

The message is therefore very clear, and a call is made to the urgent need to attract young professionals to diversify their areas of influence and consider other opportunities in all areas of influence of pharmaceutical practice and science.

Additionally, all programs (from both courses and pharmacy/pharmaceutical sciences degrees) need to be revised to understand if they are fit for purpose so that the pharmacist may actively contribute to the growing societal needs.

Foundation Training and Early Career Development

With this second WDG, the objective is the promotion of continuous training infrastructures in place for the early post-graduation years of the pharmaceutical workforce as a basis for consolidating initial education and training and, at the same time, catalyzing the progress of the novice graduated workforce towards advanced practice.

This step is of fundamental importance, given the existing disparities among basic training in the pharmaceutical workforce. This will require the proper engagement of Academia with Professional Organizations, along with the cooperation of the individuals who will have to assume a pro-active approach in enriching their post-registration knowledge.

Clear drivers and potential indicators for this development goal are described by FIP in their public reflection paper (FIP, 2016b), and they are:

- To *create clear and purposeful education and training pathways/programs to support post-registration (post-graduation) foundation training (clinical practice and pharmaceutical science areas)* (FIP, 2016b);
- To *develop early-career maps and frameworks to support a seamless transition into early career practice and towards advanced practice* (FIP, 2016b);

- To *develop structured approaches to early career mentoring systems to support novice practitioners to engage with peers and preceptors (in clinical practice and pharmaceutical science areas across the pharmaceutical workforce)* (FIP, 2016b).

This WDG is articulated with the expected professional development occurring after the initial training. Concrete planning and pathways need to be easily identified by the workforce in order to understand the options they must meaningfully contribute to the development of the pharmacist or pharmaceutical scientist profession.

Quality Assurance

This refers to the existence of transparent, contemporary and innovative processes that allow for the quality assurance of needs-based education and training systems (FIP, 2016b). This is important and considered essential, to:

- *Ensure the quality of the workforce by quality assuring the continuous development and the delivery of adequate and appropriate education and training; quality assurance needs to address academic and institutional infrastructure in order to deliver the required needs and competency-based education and training* (FIP, 2016b).
- *Establish standards-based global guidance for quality assurance of pharmacy and pharmaceutical science education in the context of local needs and practice* (FIP, 2016b).
- *Implement fair, effective and transparent policies and procedures for quality assurance of pharmacy and pharmaceutical science education and training* (FIP, 2016b).
- *Define critical stakeholder input on the development of adequate education and training and fair and effective policies, including necessary student input* (FIP, 2016b).

These are perhaps the most difficult objectives to implement from the Academic Cluster of WDGs because they refer to political, economic and scientific aspects that are in many countries regulated by other parties outside Universities, Schools and Professional Organizations.

Transparent and coherent evaluation of curricular content is necessary to ensure all degrees meet educational standards (Law et al., 2019). The content and composition of curricula are often shaped by national accreditation standards set by the government's education agencies (when these agencies are enforced), national pharmacy professional associations or regulators, or both (Law et al., 2019).

As mentioned by Law et al. (2019) *in addition to adhering to national standards, curricular development in some schools is also influenced by international accreditation standards sought by the schools themselves.*

This means that for that quality assurance needs to be satisfied, proper dialogue needs to be established with different stakeholders, namely Governmental stakeholders who provide, in many Countries, funding and are responsible for the agencies regulating the quality assurance of Universities and Schools.

In the situation that formal accreditation institutions or processes are not in place, there is the need to might have to rely on institutional quality assurance mechanisms, educational research, competency frameworks, and global pharmacy education organizations to evaluate their curricular content (Law et al., 2019), establishing meaningful partnerships if needed in order to achieve these objectives.

THE TIPPING POINT: THE 2016 NANJING STATEMENTS

With the intent of shaping the academic education of pharmacists and pharmaceutical scientists, and by capturing the views of many academic institutions and stakeholders, FIP catalyzed the Global Conference on Pharmacy & Pharmaceutical Sciences Education held in the city of Nanjing (Popular Republic of China) in November 2016, aiming to adopt three key documents that would serve as guidance for the development of the pharmaceutical workforce creating standards across the globe.

Before adoption and discussion at the Conference "The Nanjing Statements", as they would become known, underwent extensive consultation and validation processes before, during and after the Global Conference. There were 3 validation phases, with the first draft proposal including a total of 80 statements grouped into eight clusters (FIP, 2017).

During Validation Phase I, where the 80 statements were open to public consultation before the Conference, a total of 3216 comments covering 22 countries and territories were received, scrutinized and compiled, and a designated working group compiled a new proposal of 70 statements (FIP, 2017).

A second Validation Phase (II) was initiated in November 2016 during the Conference where a live vote took place by 36 delegations of 37 countries. From the 70 statements voted, 64 reached more than 80% agreement at the Global Conference (FIP, 2017).

In Validation Phase III, an attempt to clarify the reasons behind not reaching a significant consensus on 6 statements was conducted via online interaction. According to FIP, in this third validation phase, *the Working Group on Statements kept one, consolidate four into two and eliminated one of the statements* (FIP, 2017).

There is clearly a before and after the Global Conference in Nanjing. Not only this raised, for the first time, a broad dialogue on the education of pharmacists, but it also allowed different countries, territories, and regions to have a saying in what they expect from their pharmacists as foundational building health professionals of their Societies.

The final version of the Nanjing Statements includes 67 statements resulting from a large consensus and provide a clear steer in terms of the international expectations regarding education and professional training of professionals, prepared to deal with the exciting future ahead. This is also a global acknowledgment that there is a great disparity between the worldwide format of courses and post-graduate training and these are not generally adapted to the challenges to come, and if nothing changes there is the risk that the pharmacy professionals will not contribute actively to the local needs of the community they are working with.

It's acknowledged that no meaningful change is possible without time for stakeholders to get involved and foundational changes occur that allow for better funding or allocation of resources. Additionally, there is also the need to adjust mentalities, perceptions, and training of mentors and academics so that this unified vision may permeate all levels of education.

The final version of the statements distributes the statements over 8 different clusters:

1. Shared Global Vision.
2. Professional Skills Mix.
3. Recruitment of Students.
4. Foundation Training and Leadership.
5. Experiential Education.
6. Resources and Academic Staff.
7. Quality Assurance.
8. Continuing Professional Development.

The following tables were taken from official FIP documentation and reflect not only the 8 clusters but also the 67 statements that substantiate each cluster.

Cluster 1 – Shared Global Vision

In this Cluster (Table 1), the position of the pharmaceutical workforce is put in the context of the priorities and resources of the countries or regions.

Hopefully, this local alignment will also allow for the global broader alignment of a vision for the role of the pharmacist as a catalyst for better health for the populations. It's reinforced the need for foundational education of pharmacists in basic sciences, while at the same time it is very clearly stated that students must gain competencies in professional values, ethics and professionalism.

Academy needs also to be vigilant of the trends in science and profession so that the curricula are updated regularly and ebbed with the latest state of the art.

Table 1. Cluster 1 – Shared Global Vision

Cluster 1	Shared Global Vision
Description of the cluster:	A shared global vision promotes workforce development in the context of pharmaceutical education and training. This global vision should help professional leadership bodies, educators and regulators in developing a national or regional vision based on the priorities and resources of the country or region, aiming to develop new medicines and improving their use for better health.
1.1	Workforce planning, at national and local levels, should include the roles of all relevant personnel, (e.g. pharmacy technicians/assistants, generalist pharmacists, specialists, advanced practitioners, and pharmaceutical scientists) enough to meet local health needs as part of the health care system.
1.2	The education and training of pharmacists should have an underlying foundation in both the physical and biological sciences enough to prepare the student for current and future practice.
1.3	Schools[1] should teach students so they can attain competencies in professional values, ethics, and professionalism by graduation in order to improve the responsible use of medicines, their discovery, development, manufacturing and distribution.
1.4	Schools should ensure that the needs and future trends in health care delivery, advancement in the profession, the pharmaceutical industry and education are considered to develop and update the curriculum.
1.5	Schools should promote the message that pharmacists are patient advocates and care providers who provide/facilitate efficient access to quality medicines with the goal of helping patients make the best use of their medicines.
1.6	Academic staff should add to the evidence that pharmacists can improve the responsible use of medicines to improve effectiveness, safety and efficient use of limited resources and should convey to the students the skills to achieve this.
1.7	All pharmacists and academic staff should be encouraged to participate in scholarly activity to generate new knowledge in their area of expertise.
1.8	Pharmacists should be champions for good health and wellness promotion, preventive medicine and holistic patient management. Pharmacists must undertake this through an economic, social, cultural and ethical perspective.

(FIP, 2017)

Source: The table was copied from "The Nanjing Statements 2017" by the International Pharmaceutical Federation (FIP) 1 – In this document, schools are defined as "Schools of Pharmacy and/or Pharmaceutical Sciences"

Most importantly, all staff – emphasis in all – working in the education of pharmacists need to be aware of the mission and relevance of the pharmacist as a healthcare provider so that this spirit is transmitted to students from the early stages of their training.

Cluster 2 – Professional Skills Mix

As presented in Table 2, pro-active training in professional skills needs to be pursued by pharmacists working in all settings.

Again, emphasis is given to the need of ensuring a proper balance between science and practice and taught biomedical sciences. Interestingly, and for the first time, the introduction of regulatory sciences in the curricula is discussed.

Additionally, besides basic sciences, clinical, social and administrative sciences appear fundamental when they support learning about patients and their use of medicines.

Collaborative and cross-disciplinary learning are cornerstones of a progressive way of integrating several professional skills in graduation, post-graduation and professional training.

Emphasis is also given to the lifelong learning and critical thinking as core competencies of pharmacists and pharmaceutical scientists.

Cluster 3 – Recruitment of Students

As presented in Table 3, there are also some recommendations regarding the recruitment of students.

Nevertheless, in many countries or regions, these are difficult to implement given the differences in access to a University degree.

Cluster 4 – Foundation Training and Leadership

Cluster 4 (Table 4) sets the scene for the development of leadership in students and new graduates in both pharmacy and pharmaceutical sciences.

The concept of clinical competency and the need for assessment throughout their courses so that the extent of the learning of these skills is known and corrected in case it is considered deficient.

Skills in communication, entrepreneurship, and leadership should be nested in the learnings taught in schools so that the workforce is prepared for the competitive future ahead.

Table 2. Cluster 2 – Professional Skills Mix

Cluster 2	Professional Skills Mix
Description of the cluster:	Pharmacists in all settings and pharmaceutical scientists need competence, skills, knowledge, and attitudes to meet the needs of the public and interact with other health care professionals.
2.1	The proper balance of science and practice should be established and taught biomedical sciences, including pathophysiology, pharmacology, and pharmacotherapy should be distributed throughout the curriculum and should be taught in the context of patients and medicines.
2.2	Aspects of pharmaceutical chemistry, pharmaceutical technology, and pharmaceutical analysis should be included in the curriculum to present the processes related to the development, production and registration of medicinal products. Students should be taught both basic pharmaceutical sciences and the use of medicines in the context of patient care.
2.3	Pharmaceutical regulatory sciences should be included as part of the curriculum to provide knowledge and skills to students relevant to ensure the quality and safety of medicines and appropriate professional practice.
2.4	Besides the basic sciences, clinical, social, and administrative sciences are fundamental when they support learning about patients and their use of medicines.
2.5	Training and education in ethical competence should be explicitly described as a core competency and as part of the professionalism of the pharmacist in scientific and clinical practice.
2.6	Students must develop the knowledge and skills to critically assess scientific evidence, including that which applies to patient care and population health.
2.7	Graduate education and training for the pharmaceutical workforce should include opportunities for cross-disciplinary learning.
2.8	Professional communication, documentation, lifelong learning, and critical thinking should be the core competencies of pharmacists and pharmaceutical scientists.
2.9	Students should have the ability and opportunity to learn to apply the scientific knowledge that is taught in the classroom in any field within the profession.
2.10	Pharmaceutical science courses will have a laboratory component to enhance students' scientific skills.
2.11	Pharmacists should learn to work collaboratively with other health care professionals and scientists in medical, scientific and social fields.

(FIP, 2017)

Source: This Table was taken from "The Nanjing Statements 2017" by the International Pharmaceutical Federation (FIP)

Cluster 5 – Experimental Education

Cluster 5 is an inspiration for every educator. It provides the grounds for programs to be based on problem-solving processes and in the development of critical thinking.

This allows students to be better prepared for real-life settings and in direct contact with patients. The culture of risk assessment, risk management, and patient safety is to be communicated clearly as an objective for a pharmacist when practicing in different settings and is an integrant part of the education that should be provided to each professional.

Table 3. Cluster 3 – Recruitment of Students

Cluster 3	Recruitment of Students
Description of the cluster:	Recruiting students who have a profile that fits the requirements of the school and is aligned with the profile of pharmacists desired for the country.
3.1	Admissions practices should consider the value of a diverse student body reflecting regional population characteristics.
3.2	Students entering a school should have a strong scientific background, evidence of good academic performance, and demonstrate good social and emotional skills.

(FIP, 2017)

Source: This Table was taken from "The Nanjing Statements 2017" by the International Pharmaceutical Federation (FIP)

Table 4. Cluster 4 – Foundation Training and Leadership

Cluster 4	Foundation Training and Leadership
Description of the cluster:	Foundation training includes the process of education and leadership development for students and new graduates in pharmacy and the pharmaceutical sciences with a priority on developing the next generation of clinical, scientific, academic and professional leaders.
4.1	There is a common scientific core for both pharmacists and pharmaceutical scientists, but the context for learning and teaching is different.
4.2	Students should understand the social determinants of health.
4.3	Clinical competency should be assessed at relevant stages and assessment of student learning must determine the extent to which students can effectively apply the knowledge taught in practice.
4.4	Assessment of student learning should include the ability for independent and self-directed learning that is necessary for continuing professional development after graduation.
4.5	Pharmaceutical scientists and pharmacists should gain skills in interpersonal communication and teamwork.
4.6	Schools should prepare students to be future mentors, supervisors, preceptors, and leaders. This includes promoting a culture of peer support and knowledge sharing among students and encouraging students to mentor younger students.

(FIP, 2017)

Source: This Table was taken from "The Nanjing Statements 2017" by the International Pharmaceutical Federation (FIP)

Table 5. Cluster 5 – Experiential Education

Cluster 5	Experiential Education
Description of the cluster:	Experiential education programs are where students incrementally develop their pharmacy practice and science skills in a wide variety of real-life settings.
5.1	Experiential education should foster the development of critical thinking and problem-solving processes relative to drug discovery and medicine use.
5.2	Students should have the opportunity to reflect on the clinical learning experience through patient case presentations, and development and discussions of patient notes/ pharmaceutical care plans.
5.3	Pharmacy students should participate in direct patient care experiences in hospital and community practice settings and other practice experiences defined by local needs for pharmacists.
5.4	Students should be provided with supervised laboratory and clinical experience throughout the curriculum, including demonstrations and simulations.
5.5	Students should have the opportunity to learn to apply the clinical and pharmaceutical knowledge that is taught in the classroom in practical settings by working under the supervision of a faculty member or volunteer preceptor with patients and other healthcare professionals and with other scientists.
5.6	Students should have the opportunity to participate in internships/rotations with appropriate supervision and guidance, based on mutually determined learning objectives.
5.7	Students should have opportunities to learn in a wide array of practice environments, including caring for a diverse group of patients in various cultural and health state environments.
5.8	Non-traditional settings (e.g. regulatory, industrial, non-governmental organizations) are appropriate environments for selective experiential education internships/ rotations.
5.9	The culture of risk assessment, risk management, and patient safety should be communicated clearly as an objective for a pharmacist when practicing in different settings.
5.10	Students should demonstrate the ability and the right attitude to follow confidentiality policies.
5.11	Preceptors should be provided with opportunities to contribute to curricular decision-making, assessment, and strategic activities.

(FIP, 2017)

Source: This Table was taken from "The Nanjing Statements 2017" by the International Pharmaceutical Federation (FIP)

The diversity of experiences acquired in non-traditional settings is also encouraged as an integral part of an educational program.

Table 6. Cluster 6 – Resources and Academic Staff

Cluster 6	Resources and Academic Staff
Description of the cluster:	Resources and academic staff refer to equipment, finances, technology, and human resources needed to properly prepare pharmacists and pharmaceutical scientists.
6.1	Schools should allocate resources to demonstrate opportunities and disciplines available to both pharmacists and pharmaceutical scientists.
6.2	Financial resources (public funding, contributions from students, and other sources) should enable the objectives of pharmaceutical education and training to be met.
6.3	The facilities and equipment for practice and science laboratory work should be up to date, in good condition, and in enough quantity to allow learners to benefit from practical learning.
6.4	Required educational resources and supporting technologies should be available to students in the school.
6.5	A safe environment should be provided for faculty staff and learners.
6.6	Academic staff should have academic or professional experience that supports their main areas of teaching and research.
6.7	Academic staff should demonstrate active participation in sharing their knowledge and promoting collaboration with colleagues in their field (and other fields) at a national and international level.
6.8	The teaching performance of academic staff should be taken into consideration for their academic advancement.
6.9	Academic staff should demonstrate that they continuously update their teaching material to ensure relevance to contemporary aspects and support future developments.
6.10	Active learning techniques should be used in the classroom by academic staff.
6.11	All academic staff should engage in continuing professional development that is relevant to their work and responsibilities.
6.12	Academic staff at schools should collaborate with preceptors and experiential learning sites to assure quality learning.
6.13	All academic staff should have opportunities to contribute to curricular decision-making.
6.14	The school should support and promote the academic staff, preceptors, students, and administrators to engage in professional activities with other health sectors.
6.15	The school should support and promote the participation of academic staff, preceptors, students, and administrators in national and international activities of pharmacy and related experiences.

(FIP, 2017)

Source: This Table was taken from "The Nanjing Statements 2017" by the International Pharmaceutical Federation (FIP)

Table 7. Cluster 7 – Quality Assurance

Cluster 7	Quality Assurance
Description of the cluster:	Quality assurance refers to the key aspects and mechanisms to identify opportunities for and make improvement in pharmacy and pharmaceutical sciences education to ensure a good, sustainable performance and suitable competencies of the future workforce.
7.1	A quality improvement program should be in place at the school and university, and examples of specific improvement should be demonstrated periodically.
7.2	Metrics should exist to measure, monitor, manage, and improve the quality of the education and training provided.
7.3	Quality metrics should include feedback from students and new graduates, faculty, preceptors, and key external stakeholders, such as employers and professional bodies.
7.4	Policies and procedures support the regular review of the curriculum and allow developments in the curriculum to take place in a timely manner to keep up with the changes in the profession, technology, and society.
7.5	The pharmacy and pharmaceutical scientist degree programs should be offered at a university level and all the experiential components (placements) in clinical, industrial, and institutional settings are undertaken under the supervision of the school.
7.6	Students should have the opportunity to participate in internships/rotations with Competencies and should be assessed throughout the curriculum, not just at the end of it, and before the internship period.
7.7	A formal system of quality assurance, administered by a government or an independent agency approved by the government, should be in place and required for all schools.
7.8	The accreditation system should use published standards that have been developed and adopted with broad stakeholder involvement.
7.9	The accreditation system should use policies and procedures that ensure evaluation by appropriately qualified and experienced peers; absence of conflict of interest; confidentiality; and fair and consistent application of standards.
7.10	Quality improvement should always include a clear process for handling student concerns/ issues/complaints that is transparent so that students are informed of the progress and outcome of any concern that is raised.

(FIP, 2017)

Source: The table was copied from "The Nanjing Statements 2017" by the International Pharmaceutical Federation (FIP)

Table 8. Cluster 8 – Continuing Professional Development

Cluster 8	Continuing Professional Development
Description of the cluster:	Continuing professional development (CPD) refers to building on previous education as a pharmacist and pharmaceutical scientist.
8.1	CPD should apply both to those in the regulated professional practice and those working in unregulated professional practice, such as academia and the pharmaceutical sciences.
8.2	All members of the pharmaceutical workforce should accept a responsibility to manage their CPD.
8.3	The promotion of CPD should begin with students at the start of their education.
8.4	Schools should support CPD for graduate professionals to prepare them for advanced practice roles.

(FIP, 2017)

Source: This Table was taken from "The Nanjing Statements 2017" by the International Pharmaceutical Federation (FIP)

Cluster 6 – Resources and Academic Staff

As the descriptor of the Cluster mentions (Table 6), in this cluster *resources and academic staff refer to equipment, finances, technology and human resources needed to properly prepare pharmacists and pharmaceutical scientists* (FIP, 2017) and this makes this cluster aspirational only in some of the countries or territories.

It's also one of the hardest clusters to implement given the dependence on funding. Nevertheless, the call for active learning techniques is very clear and these can be transversally applied without much equipment, only by providing proper training to academic staff.

Cluster 7 – Quality Assurance

As previously mentioned, WDG number 3 under the Academic Cluster is all about Quality Assurance (Table 7), detailing how every country and region should have *transparent, contemporary and innovative processes for the quality assurance of needs-based education and training systems* (Law et al., 2019).

Cluster 8 – Continuing Professional Development

This last cluster reiterates the importance of the continuous development of the workforce (Table 8) building on previous education and training.

It is perhaps one of the most fundamental concepts that need to be properly implemented in each country or region.

Competency-based education can prepare a pharmacist for the beginning of its professional life; however, no unique pharmaceutical education program can ensure all the scientific and social skills that a pharmacist will need throughout its career.

To achieve this kind of preparation it is necessary to combine the foundations of a good pre-graduation program along with in-service training, work experience, and lifetime knowledge acquisition. For pharmacists, education is a continuum.

The use of the same successful educational strategies and objective-driven outcome approaches employed for pre-graduation knowledge acquisition should be continued and improved along with the pharmacist career (Rouse, 2004).

As previously mentioned, these statements work as a reminder of the goals for the education of pharmacists worldwide.

The uptake of these goals by stakeholders is critical for the success of this initiative. Law et al., in one of the very few existing published manuscripts about the Nanjing Statements, rightly mention the importance of these statements being interiorized by academic administrators and leaders (Law et al., 2019). Each of the clusters previously presented address multiple challenges and provide educational roadmaps that may guide the transformational change expected in the pharmaceutical workforce.

The same authors (Law et al., 2019) mention that a self-assessment tool is being validated by FIP in collaboration with other stakeholders, so that each school may evaluate the level of implementation of the Nanjing Statements and therefore determine the areas requiring further investment and improvement in order to reach the goals (Law et al., 2019).

The scarcity of publications on the subject, and the slow uptake of these changes, currently do not allow for an in-depth analysis of the impact of these statements.

MEETING THE CHALLENGE AND EMBRACING THE CHANGE

As it is evident from the considerations above, FIP is heavily involved in the process of creating a vision for the future of the Pharmacy and Pharmaceutical Sciences, and this is a positive thing. FIP is also committed to providing all the appropriate tools to its members so that they can apply the Nanjing Statements at a local level.

However, both WHO and UNESCO are also involved in the process, as in 2008 the three organizations worked in tandem in what would be known as *The WHO UNESCO FIP Pharmacy Education and Taskforce* (Anderson et al., 2008) declaring that the role of the pharmacist evolved as a professional that produced and distributed medicines, to become the specialist of medicines in multidisciplinary healthcare teams (Anderson et al., 2008).

It also reinforces that in the context of developing countries the pharmacy is often the most accessible or even the only point of access to obtain healthcare advice and services for the majority of citizens (Anderson et al., 2009).

The purpose of the Pharmacy Education Taskforce is to *oversee the implementation of the 2008–2010 Pharmacy Education Action Plan, identify resources and serve as a connection for stakeholders*. The Action Plan is an *initiative to develop evidence-based guidelines and frameworks that will facilitate the development of pharmacy education*. The aim of this Action Plan is *to enable the sustainability of a pharmacy workforce, advocating for needs-based pharmacy education development. Needs-based education means that education is determined locally by evaluating the services required, the competencies needed to provide such services, and using that to plan education which would support the development of such competencies* (Figure 1) (Manasse, Brock, & Gal, 2009).

Figure 1. WHO UNESCO FIP Pharmacy Education Taskforce Action Plan
(Manasse et al., 2009)
Source: Adapted from the 4th Annual Global Pharmacy Education Consultation Report

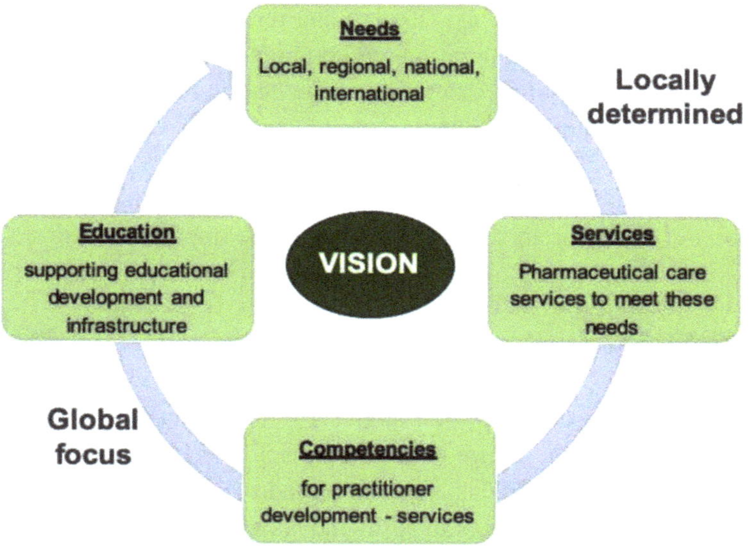

Due to their knowledge of medicines and clinical therapy, pharmacists are uniquely placed for specialized tasks in the healthcare network and should be trained to perform clinical management and laboratory diagnosis functions. It is, therefore, necessary to train and provide high standards of education to these professionals in order to prepare them for such roles.

Recognizing that healthcare needs can vary across geography and culture, stakeholders in pharmacy education and global health have reached a unanimous agreement that pharmacy education should be driven by quality and targeted at healthcare needs, the services needed to meet these needs, the skills necessary to provide these services and the education necessary to ensure these skills.

At the student level, the International Pharmaceutical Students' Federation (IPSF) also follows the same line of thought and through the events and educational activities they organize, such as the "Clinical Skills Event", "Patient Counseling Event", "Public Health Camps" and "Trainers Development Camp", this organization is helping to meet the WDGs and provide students with many of the skills present in the Nanjing Statements and that Academy is not yet able to meet.

IPSF, after the publication of the Nanjing Statements and WDGs, conducted an inquiry to determine if students thought these goals were feasible in their country and if they agreed that students should play an active role in these discussions and the same documents would create a change worldwide. Unfortunately, the results have not been shared.

At European Union level we can say that Education is more uniform due to directives such as Directive 2005/36/EC Recognition of Professional Qualifications in Practice which despite having as main objective the promotion of mobility of professionals between the Member States, has led to certain foundational disciplines being taught in all Member States and that basic training is uniform or close to being the same. Bologna's process has also contributed to this greater standardization and assurance that students have similar basic education. The Bologna Process is a strictly intergovernmental initiative and aims to create a Common European Higher Education Area.

At the European level, there are also more organizations interested in education such as the EAFP- European Association of Faculties of Pharmacy that has been involved in projects such as PHARMINE: Pharmacy Education in Europe (2008-2010), PHAR-QA: Quality Assurance in European Pharmacy Education and Training (2012-2016) and PHAR-IN: Competencies for Industrial pharmacy in biotechnology (2014-2016).

There is also the role of EUFEPS (European Federation for Pharmaceutical Sciences), which also provides educational activities more directed to the Pharmaceutical Sciences. They also organize a Congress in collaboration with FIP on Pharmaceutical Sciences.

At the student level, there is the EPSA- European Pharmaceutical Students' Association that in addition to providing the most varied activities such as Mentoring Project, EPSA Training Project, High-quality program in its events, webinars, public health campaigns also have a strong political nature in order to produce various opinion statements and positions. The most important ones for Education were: Position

Paper on Soft-Skills, Joint Policy Paper on Interprofessional Education, Position Paper on Pharmaceutical Care in the Curriculum in conjunction with the EAFP.

Also, in the journal publications setting the young pharmacist's community has been actively participating in the evolution of pharmacy education worldwide with the existence of the peer-reviewed Medline-indexed journal, Journal of Young Pharmacists. A review article entitled "The changing face of pharmacy practice and the need for a new model of pharmacy education" highlighted that pharmacy schools should develop an education curriculum that accompanies the evolving roles of the pharmaceutical profession (Toklu & Hussain, 2013).

The evolving role of the pharmacy profession is a demanding challenge that mandates that the educational institutes must intervene with competent curricula. Education must ensure the acquisition of crucial tools enabling the pharmacy professionals for critical thinking, problem-solving skills, and pharmacotherapeutic decisions (Toklu & Hussain, 2013).

CONCLUSION

The pharmaceutical workforce of the future must be educated to be able to create, transfer, and also to apply new knowledge based on the evolution of science in the pharmaceutical, social, and clinical settings; this will only be possible by providing students and professionals with the tools to understand science, research, and soft-skills, allowing them to cooperate with all other health professionals, to ultimately achieving the main goal which is to boost the well-being of the society and global community by improving the health of each individual (Toklu & Hussain, 2013).

REFERENCES

Anderson, C., Bates, I., Beck, D., Brock, T., Futter, B., Mercer, H., … Yonemura, A. (2008). The WHO UNESCO FIP Pharmacy Education Taskforce: Enabling concerted and collective global action. *American Journal of Pharmaceutical Education*. doi:10.5688/aj7206127

Anderson, C., Bates, I., Beck, D., Brock, T. P., Futter, B., Mercer, H., Rouse, M., Whitmarsh, S., Wuliji, T., & Yonemura, A. (2009). The WHO UNESCO FIP Pharmacy Education Taskforce. *Human Resources for Health*, *7*(1), 45. Advance online publication. doi:10.1186/1478-4491-7-45 PMID:19500351

FIP. (2008). *FIP's Vision, Mission and Strategic Plan*. Retrieved from https://www.fip.org/files/fip/strategic plan no annexes.pdf

FIP. (2016a). *Global Vision for Education and Workforce Presented at the global conference on pharmacy and Pharmaceutical sciences education Nanjing Declaration Global Vision for a Global Pharmaceutical Workforce by Advancing Practice and Science through Transformative*. Retrieved from https://www.fip.org/files/fip/PharmacyEducation/2016_report/2016-11-Education-workforce-global-vision.pdf

FIP. (2016b). *Pharmaceutical Workforce Development Goals*. Retrieved from https://www.fip.org/files/content/priority-areas/workforce/wdgs-online-version.pdf

FIP. (2017). *Nanjing Statements*. Retrieved from https://www.fip.org/files/content/priority-areas/workforce/nanjing-statements.pdf

FIP. (2019). *The FIP Workforce Transformation Programme (WTP)*. Retrieved from https://www.fip.org/files/fip/PharmacyEducation/2019/FIP-WTP-program-web.pdf

Law, M., Bader, L., Uzman, N., Williams, A., & Bates, I. (2019). *The FIP Nanjing Statements: Shaping global pharmacy and pharmaceutical sciences education. In Research in Social and Administrative Pharmacy*. Elsevier Inc., doi:10.1016/j.sapharm.2019.03.013

Manasse, H. R., Brock, T., & Gal, D. (2009). *WHO UNESCO FIP Pharmacy Education Taskforce 4th Annual Global Pharmacy Education Consultation Report?* Retrieved from www.fip.org/education

Rouse, M. J. (2004). Continuing Professional Development in Pharmacy. *The Journal of Pharmacy Technology*, *20*(5), 303–306. doi:10.1177/875512250402000509

Toklu, H. Z., & Hussain, A. (2013). The changing face of pharmacy practice and the need for a new model of pharmacy education. *Journal of Young Pharmacists*. E-Flow Medknow Publications. doi:10.1016/j.jyp.2012.09.001

United Nations. (2019). *Transforming our world: The 2030 agenda for sustainable development United Nations transforming our world: The 2030 agenda for sustainable development*. Retrieved from https://sustainabledevelopment.un.org/content/documents/21252030 Agenda for Sustainable Development web.pdf

ENDNOTE

1 The FIP Workforce Transformation Programme (WTP) defines "Pharmaceutical Workforce" as the whole of the pharmacy related workforce (e.g. registered pharmacist practitioners, pharmaceutical scientists, pharmacy technicians and other pharmacy support workforce cadres, pre-service students/trainees) working in a diversity of settings (e.g. community, hospital, research and development, industry, military, regulatory, academia and other sectors) with a diversity of scopes of practice.

Chapter 3
Teaching and Learning Methods for Drug Information

Fernando Fernandez-Llimos
Faculty of Pharmacy, University of Porto, Portugal

Helena H. Borba
Department of Pharmacy, Federal University of Paraná, Brazil

Antonio M. Mendes
Pharmaceutical Sciences Program, Federal University of Paraná, Brazil

Roberto Pontarolo
Department of Pharmacy, Federal University of Paraná, Brazil

Fernanda S. Tonin
Pharmaceutical Sciences Program, Federal University of Paraná, Brazil

ABSTRACT

Healthcare professionals, especially pharmacists, are constantly involved with drug information and should be able to properly select resources and keep updated on new literature and new tools to address a variety of drug information requests. The provision of accurate in-depth drug information requires the development of drug information skills through both didactic and experiential training programs. Considering the complexity of the drug information field and the expanding roles of pharmacists as information resources, this chapter will briefly introduce the main concepts of drug information and discuss the potential methods and challenges for teaching this subject while matching the variety of learning styles.

DOI: 10.4018/978-1-7998-4486-0.ch003

INTRODUCTION

The Role of the Pharmacist in Drug Information

The concept of 'information' is used in almost every scientific discipline within its own different contexts. In healthcare, 'information' may be defined as the provision of unbiased, evidence-based, and critically evaluated data and experiences (Bernknopf et al., 2009; Mononen et al., 2018).

The access to the most relevant, updated, user-specific, and objective information is paramount to make appropriate decisions (e.g. prescription, dispensing, and use of drugs), and to inform, underpin, or shape scientific research (Sharp, Bodenreider, & Wacholder, 2008).

In the early 1960s, the combination of terms 'drug information', 'center', and 'specialist' was first employed to describe a distinct practice area of Pharmacy (Malone, Kier, Stanovich, & Malone, 2014; Walton, 2006). The University of Kentucky in the United States of America set the first 'drug information center', aiming at providing patient-specific drug information, assess adverse drug reaction information, and guide student and healthcare professionals education and training (Rosenberg, Koumis, Nathan, Cicero, & McGuire, 2004; Tietze, 2012).

The pharmacist was usually considered the 'drug information specialist' or 'drug consultant' that had enough expertise and knowledge to retrieve, select, evaluate, and disseminate information towards a specific drug-related question.

This continuous support of rational therapeutic selections contributed towards better patient care and allowed the pharmacist to further integrate the multidisciplinary healthcare team (Amerson & Wallingford, 1983; Malone, et al., 2014).

Shortly after, several other 'drug information centers' were created in the United States of America, with more than 50 pharmacist-operated centers during the 1970s (Amerson & Wallingford, 1983; Rosenberg, et al., 2004). At this time, different approaches were developed to provide drug information services, including hospitals' decentralized pharmacists, clinical consultation services, and regional center for a specific geographic area (Amundstuen Reppe, Spigset, & Schjott, 2016).

Consequently, there was significant growth in the 'clinical pharmacy movement', mostly because of the acceptance of the clinical pharmacist role in patients care, the need for quick access to drug information, and the perceived ability of pharmacists to interpret conflicting therapeutic information (American Pharmacists Association, 2007).

However, in recent years, health systems in both developed and developing countries faced the challenges of financial constraints, a high prevalence of non-communicable diseases, and an increase in problems related to pharmacotherapy and morbidity and mortality associated with drug use.

These changes led to the closure of some drug information centers and significantly impacted on clinical pharmacy model and in 'pharmacy' as a profession (Iwanowicz, Marciniak, & Zeolla, 2006; World Health Organization (WHO), 1996, 1997). Still, the provision of drug information is as important today as at the beginning of the drug information concept, being an integral pharmacist responsibility that represents a core standard of the profession and also embodies numerous educational outcomes within the pharmacy curricula (Bernknopf, et al., 2009; Gonzalez et al., 2019).

According to the World Health Organization (WHO), pharmacists have a vital role to play in drug therapy management and should be more involved in solving healthcare problems. This includes being able to provide evidence-based recommendations, which may support clinical practices, enhance the quality of patient care, improve patients' outcomes, and ensure the rational use of resources (World Health Organization (WHO), 1996, 1997).

In a recent report of the ASHP Foundation, one of the 2015 initiatives is to continuously increase the extent to which health-system pharmacists apply evidence-based methods to improve medication therapies (S. Ghaibi, Ipema, Gabay, & American Society of Health-System, 2015; Manasse, 2005).

The pharmacist must have skills in oral and written communication domains to effectively provide drug information, being able to:

1. Anticipate and objectively evaluate the drug information needs of patients and other healthcare professionals.
2. Obtain appropriate and complete background information for responding to any drug information request.
3. Use a systematic and stepwise approach to address drug information needs by searching, retrieving, and critically evaluating the literature (i.e. assessment of study design, statistics, bias, limitations, and applicability).
4. Appropriately synthesize, communicate, document, disseminate, and apply pertinent information to each situation.

Consequently, a reorientation of pharmacy education is necessary. Curriculum modifications and instructional strategies should be considered to facilitate learning outcomes, in terms of the knowledge and skills needed for drug information practice.

Pharmacists should be involved in expanded patient care responsibilities, which require adequate knowledge, communication skills, problem-solving capabilities, critical-thinking abilities, and decision-making skills (AlHaqwi, Kuntze, & van der Molen, 2014; Nathan, 2013).

BACKGROUND

Information Literacy

The recent advances in communication technology and internet access allowed a faster and broader dissemination of information worldwide. More than 1,000,000 biomedical journal articles are published annually, most of them with online access (Berland et al., 2001; Iwanowicz, et al., 2006), which turns impossible to healthcare professionals to keep up-to-date with the most reliable evidence.

This 'paradox of the information' reflects the apparent contradiction that the more information we have access to, the more difficult is to use it (Alper et al., 2004; Davies & Harrison, 2007; Eysenbach, Powell, Kuss, & Sa, 2002).

The definition of the term 'information literacy' has been articulated by a range of models and terminology developed by both academics and librarians. According to the American Library Association (ALA), 'information literacy' is the ability to recognize when information is needed, then to locate and evaluate the appropriate information, and finally to use it effectively and responsibly (ALA Presidential Committee on Information Literacy, 1989).

Because information now comes in many different formats, both printed and electronically, and its quality varies enormously, healthcare professionals need to develop the cognitive and transferable skills to be able to work efficiently with information. This includes an understanding, amongst others, of the resources available, how to find information and evaluate results, how to work with or exploit results, ethical and responsible use, and how to communicate or share findings (ALA Presidential Committee on Information Literacy, 1989; Eisenberg, 2008; Hersh et al., 2014).

In practical terms, pharmacists need full-access to information about drugs including formulation, indications, and contraindications for use, therapeutic alternatives, dosing and regimen, drug-interactions, side-effects, adverse events, clinical features, and costs (Dickinson, Raynor, Knapp, & MacDonald, 2017; Gonzalez-Gonzalez et al., 2007).

Drug Information Sources

Primary, Secondary and Tertiary Sources

The format in which information is available varies according to the needs of end-users. Traditionally, information resources were classified accordingly to their physical format in primary, secondary, and tertiary.

Primary sources were those providing original data, usually published as printed material (e.g. articles, reports, and journals).

Secondary sources were those used to guide the review of primary literature (e.g. abstract compilations, microfiches, and databases) and tertiary sources were those printed 'processed information' (e.g. books) (Kier & Goldwire, 2018).

Nonetheless, with the development of information technologies and the global access to any online information, sources are now classified according to the originality of the information and the periodicity of the publication.

The periodicity of publication refers not only to standardized periods of publication (e.g. weekly, annually) but also to the content characteristics. To be periodical, an information source needs to provide different contents at each new edition; differently to the update of a non-periodical source which includes the addition of some new content together with the old one.

Primary sources are periodical publications that provide original material, being useful for research, education, and current awareness. This source typically consists of journal articles or reports (e.g. original research, clinical trials, pharmacological research, opinions) (S Ghaibi, Ipema, & Gabay, 2015; Miranda, Vercellesi, & Bruno, 2004), and usually provides the most up-to-date information that is quickly published. On the other hand, this information can be immature, that is, not sufficiently contrasted with other data.

Secondary sources are more difficult to define because interpretations vary as to what exactly they are, but, as definition, they include non-original texts. That is to say, they incorporate material from primary or tertiary sources. Secondary sources include indexing and abstracting systems that organize and provide easy retrieval of literature. Indexing systems include the article citation, with or without access to the abstract, and some allow access to the full-text article. On the other hand, abstracting services provide not only the citation but also the abstract and often a link to the full-text article.

Examples of these resources include MEDLINE (through PubMed, EBSCO, Ovid), Scopus, Cochrane Database of Systematic Reviews, International Pharmaceutical Abstracts (IPA). These resources have detailed and user-friendly search engines that enable literature searches on a specific topic. However, proper training is required for efficient use of these systems. The cost of secondary resources is typically based on the number of users granted access; thus, they often require a library or institutional budget to finance (Clauson, Marsh, Polen, Seamon, & Ortiz, 2007; Kier & Goldwire, 2018; Stansfield, Brunton, & Rees, 2014).

Tertiary sources are original summarized information (i.e. interpretation and conclusions) that compile and contrast the information contained mainly in primary sources. Differently from the primary sources, tertiary sources are not periodically published. Tertiary sources include textbooks, compendia, reference books, formal reports, some electronic databases (e.g. Micromedex, Up-To-Date, Dynamed).

These references often are the starting point to identify information, because they typically provide a fairly complete overview of information on a specific topic. However, their most significant limitation is the lag time for publication (American Pharmacists Association, 2007; Kier & Goldwire, 2018).

Official and Non-Official Information Sources

Information sources can also be classified accordingly to the producer of the information. A source is official when it is either produced or approved by an official regulatory body, such as regulatory agencies, or by independent scientific societies or academic groups.

Examples of these sources include Summaries of Product Characteristics (SmPCs), package leaflet, European Public Assessment Report (EPAR).

On the other hand, other sources of information, produced to aid healthcare providers and researchers are classified as unofficial (Kier & Goldwire, 2018; Stansfield, et al., 2014).

Literature Search

To find information, pharmacists and students should perform a literature search, defined as a systematic and comprehensive search of data, that can be carried out in any available source. Generally, the best method to find information includes a stepwise approach moving first through tertiary (e.g. textbooks, full-text databases, review articles), then secondary (e.g. indexing or abstracting services), and finally primary (e.g. clinical studies) literature.

This occurs because primary sources, although are published faster, can present more biased evidence, being usually of 'immediate' use. On the other hand, tertiary sources can provide more robust data, as information had sufficient time to be discussed amongst researchers. Secondary sources help to locate information whenever needed (Merigo & Nunez, 2016; Miranda, et al., 2004).

Search Engines and Information Retrieval

When searching for specific words or phrases (called 'search terms') related to a specific research topic, a search engine (e.g. Google, MEDLINE) is useful.

Different search engines often produce different results for the same topic; therefore, the use of more than one search engine is frequently recommended to improve results retrieval (Thiele, Poiro, Scalzo, & Nemergut, 2010).

One of the most known sources of information in the healthcare field is MEDLINE. The history of this system begins with MedLARS (Medical Literature Retrieval and Analysis System), the first large scale computerized biomedical bibliographic retrieval system, launched by the National Library of Medicine (NLM) in 1964.

Before that and since 1879, the NLM had published the Index Medicus, a monthly guide to medical articles of several journals, that was manually compiled. In late 1971, an online version called MEDLINE (MedLARS Online) became available for online searching.

Yet initially limited to libraries, the early system covered around 240 journals. Researchers could submit pre-programmed search tasks to librarians and obtain results on printouts. After that, methods for accessing information have notably progressed with the creation of the World Wide Web and the integration of electronic medical records, which allowed healthcare professionals to have a broader picture of patients and treatments. In 1996, a free public interface of MEDLINE was launched, called PubMed.

This database contains more than 26 million records covering biomedicine and health from 1950 to the present (Cummings, 1967; C. Dee, 2007; Lindberg, 2000).

Boolean Operators

Search engines use Boolean Logic operators (AND, OR, NOT) to help narrow results in search strategies. The operator AND is used between two or more search terms when research wants to find an article that contains both terms simultaneously.

Two search terms united by the operator OR will tell the engine that one or both terms must appear within the record. The operator NOT is used to search for results that do not contain one specific search term (Kier & Goldwire, 2018).

Search Strategies: Medline and MeSH Terms

The most efficient search will depend on the type of information that is needed. Besides, the use of search engines strives to balance usability with power and comprehensiveness.

Unlike using a typical internet search engine (e.g. Google), PubMed searching of MEDLINE is a learning skill. The multiple ways to search MEDLINE include the use of search terms combined with Boolean operators, by keywords of articles, by journal name, by author's name, by the title of articles, and also by Medical Subject Heading (MeSH) terms.

MeSH terms are a standardized vocabulary used specifically for indexing articles in MEDLINE. They are organized within MEDLINE in a 'tree structure'. This hierarchal system allows for either broad topic searches (e.g. pharmaceutical services) or more narrow searches (e.g. medication therapy management) (National Library of Medicine, 2019). Using the MeSH database to define the subject of interest is a useful way to improve the quality of the search. However, familiarity with these terms is necessary for an efficient and effective search (Chapman, 2009; Kier & Goldwire, 2018).

The limit function in MEDLINE also provides a means of filtering unwanted articles from a set of search results. The search parameters are limited according to the criteria the searcher selects. Examples of limits include language, human or animal species, review articles, latest updates, publication type, publication year (Delwiche, 2008).

Approach for Responding to Drug Information Requests

Besides knowing the differences between types of drug information sources and where to find each one of them, the pharmacist should be able to effectively respond to a drug information request.

A systematic approach for responding to drug information requests was first designed by Watanabe and collaborators in 1975, and then modified and expanded over the years (Fischer, 1980; Watanabe, McCart, Shimomura, & Kayser, 1975). The main steps that should be followed include:

Step 1: Identity of the requestor, in order to obtain complete information and perform the most appropriate response considering health literacy and professional background of the requestor;

Step 2: Define the real question and information needed, which will optimize the search process and guide the response to the request

Step 3: Obtaining complete background information, including patient's medical records if applicable

Step 4: Categorize the question according to the requestor (e.g. patient-specific, academic, healthcare professional) and type of question (e.g. related to the product, formulation, dosage/regimen/administration, therapeutic use, precautions, adverse drug event, drug interactions, pharmacokinetics, safety, and toxicity) to tailor the search strategy and selection of resources

Step 5: Perform the systematic search using the stepwise approach including as many sources as necessary

Step 6: Evaluate, interpret and combine the information from the resources used

Step 7: Disseminate the information by oral or written response according to the needs of the requestor and each situation

Step 8: Document all the process including the request, information resources used, information found, time spent on the response, and the response itself. This demonstrates accountability and justifies the value of pharmacist care
Step 9: Perform a follow-up assessment to determine the utility of the information provided

Drug Information and Evidence-Based Practice

Since the 1960s, the availability of new therapies (e.g. beta-blockers, different antibiotics) provided challenges to healthcare professionals to best make clinical decisions (Drews, 2000).

Part of the problem was solved with the creation of the drug information centers - represented by the figure of the drug information specialist - together with the development of the interfaces such as PubMed (C. R. Dee, 2007; Taine, 1963).

However, the advances in communication technology created a new concern: the extensive amounts of data daily published about new or already existing health technologies (e.g. drugs, devices, vaccines, procedures), which makes impossible to pharmacists to keep up-to-date with the most reliable evidence (Alper, et al., 2004; Davies & Harrison, 2007; Eysenbach, et al., 2002).

This scenario highlights the current demand for pharmacists to play a key role as drug information providers to healthcare professionals and society (Amundstuen Reppe, et al., 2016; Mears, 2009). The appropriate use of the best information available is an important component of the decision-making process that supports the safe and rational use of resources and represents significant cost-savings for the healthcare system.

In this context, professionals should be able to read and interpret the evidence provided by different types of studies and information sources (from clinical trials to systematic reviews with meta-analyses), grade the level of evidence in each scenario, and finally transpose these results to practice (Bansback et al., 2015; Chequeta & Lewis, 2009).

Besides, the pharmacist can serve as a resource for the formulation of therapeutic guidelines, in the coordination of adverse drug events programs, for the selection of cost-effective health technologies, in medication policy decisions (drug benefits), to solve other practice-related issues, among others (American Pharmacists Association, 2007; Bernknopf, et al., 2009).

TEACHING AND LEARNING METHODS

On a biological level, learning is a continuous process whereby neural pathways form and strength connections involving attention, storage, and retrieval of knowledge, skills, attitudes, and behaviors. The explanation of the learning process is usually grounded in two main theories (behavioral and cognitive theories), that influenced the development of further concepts in the field (e.g. constructivism, psychoanalytical approach, human approach) (Akdeniz & et al., 2016).

Behavioral learning theories focus on how behaviors are acquired, stating that the experiences and the environment shape a person's personality. According to researchers of this field, the human brain can be compared to a 'black box'. What goes into (input) and what comes out of (output) this black box can be adjusted, arranged, measured, and controlled; however, what happens inside the box is not fully elucidated. Learning takes place by establishing a connection between the stimulant (input) and the actual behavior, and that changing behavior is possible through reinforcement (Akdeniz & et al., 2016; Badyal & Singh, 2017).

Cognitive theories state that the mental processes (i.e. human mind activities to understand the events and situations going on around) are more important rather than stimulant-reaction connection in learning. Some of these activities include the perception of the stimulants coming from outside, the comparison of these stimulants to previous information, shaping new information, memorizing and remembering the gained information. Thus, cognitive theories focus on internal stimulants instead of external stimulants of learning (e.g. attention, perception, memory) (Akdeniz & et al., 2016; Badyal & Singh, 2017).

Based on these concepts, several teaching-learning theories have been developed worldwide. Some of them although interesting (e.g. the learning styles theory, the learning pyramid, the 10,000-hour rule, the digital natives theory), lack strong evidence on their real effect. One learning model that gained attention and is used in a variety of books, training models, and courses was developed by Martin M. Broadwell in 1969 as the 'four levels of competence' (Broadwell, 1969).

This model suggests that individuals are initially unaware of how little they know, or unconscious of their incompetence ('unconscious incompetence' stage). As they recognize their incompetence ('conscious incompetence' stage), they consciously acquire a skill, then consciously use it ('conscious competence' stage). Eventually, the skill can be used without it being consciously thought through, that is to say, the individual acquired unconscious competence ('unconscious competence' stage). This model also helps to understand the concept of 'cognitive bias' stated by Dunning-Kruger (the Dunning-Kruger effect) in which people mistakenly assess their cognitive ability as greater than it is (illusory superiority). Without the self-awareness of metacognition, a person cannot objectively evaluate their competence or incompetence (Pennycook, Ross, Koehler, & Fugelsang, 2017).

The means through which an individual acquires conscience and learn can be defined as modes or models of learning (e.g. by observation, imitation, trial or error, insight, collaboration). Teaching methods are principles and organized actions developed by teachers/educators to enable students to learn, aiming at maximizing knowledge acquisition (information storage and retrieval) for specific educational content (Schumacher, Englander, & Carraccio, 2013).

In this regard, knowledge is constructed, not transferred. Since it is built around information, past individual experiences, and the surrounding environment, there is no single way to achieve knowledge, although the process can be optimized. The major factors influencing this process are the organizing time and the duration of learning (retrieval strength and long-term memory), the structure/complexity of the subject to be learned (e.g. educational content), and learner's participation/engagement and feedback (Badyal & Singh, 2017; Schumacher, et al., 2013).

According to the cognitive load theory, as our sensory memory is constantly stimulated through different senses, we end up ignoring most of the inputs. In order to improve the 'coding' of information, this theory suggests focusing on the intrinsic (essential) actions while minimizing extraneous (distracting) items. Distraction minimization may be performed by the teacher (e.g. limiting extraneous images or words on slides during presentations, avoiding too deep or broadly on a given subject) and by the learner (e.g. compartmentalize other pending tasks to focus on the given activity). Once the data is obtained and processed, the learned information is stored as a 'memory'. However, not all created memories are equal.

In order to build a rich neural network for a given subject is important to have inputs from multiple different stimulating sources in different contexts (lectures, videos/podcasts, textbooks, discussions). This 'multimodal learning' model allows for abstract concepts to be linked to concrete frameworks and be reach from a person's memory in different scenarios. Besides, emotional activation plays an important role in memory construction. Passive learning is not that efficient when compared to learners that are engaged in a given topic (Leppink & van den Heuvel, 2015; Sharma, 2016).

Humans' memory has been extensively studied in the literature. The 'Ebbinghaus' forgetting curve', for instance, is a model that predicts how quickly we forget readily information over time if no attempt to retain it is made. Learners will rapidly lose memory of learned knowledge unless the information is consciously reviewed. Data suggest that humans forget around 50% of new information within an hour of learning it, and this rate can reach over 70% within one day.

Actively 'rehearsing information', a cognitive process in which information is repeated repeatedly as a possible way to learn and remember, is believed to be a major factor counteracting this temporal decline. Other suggestions to improve information retention include to space out multiple studies or practice sessions over an extended period of time or to use the 10% rule (i.e. to review material at an interval equal to 10% of the time you need to retain information) (Augustin, 2014; Azer, Guerrero, & Walsh, 2013; Oberauer & Lewandowsky, 2008).

Regarding the factors of structure/complexity of the subject to be learned, the concepts of interleaved learning and blocked practice can be applied. Interleaving is a process where students mix, or interleave, multiple subjects or topics while they study in order to improve their learning. On the other hand, blocked practice involves studying one topic very thoroughly before moving to another topic. Although this last seems 'easier' because it focuses on one single skill or competency intensively until the learner mastered it, this is not what occurs in daily practice.

In the case of Drug Information as a discipline, for instance, the student should be able to respond to patients' or professionals' requests which are usually a complex set of issues requiring several points of knowledge at the same time. Interleaving in learning allows the comparison of different concepts in different contexts. Mixing old, current, and upcoming information from a subject during the same study or practice session has a positive impact on strengthening future learning retrieval. This concept has implications for curriculum design, promoting more heterogeneous models (Badyal & Singh, 2017; Carvalho & Goldstone, 2015).

Additionally, the strategy of 'retrieval practice', in which we bring more information to our mind, can further enhance and boost learning. This is because deliberately recalling information forces learners to 'pull out' their knowledge and explore what they know. That is to say, learning should be effortful: the struggle to remember an answer can increase the retrieval strength of that information.

To achieve this, some alternatives such as test enhanced learning (e.g. quiz, oral presentations, and flashcard) can be used. Besides, the learner should adopt a growth mindset and commit to change (e.g. learn from mistakes, have a study routine, get involved with the subject) (Augustin, 2014; Kruger & Dunning, 1999).

Drug Information as an Educational Subject in Pharmacy Curricula

Pharmacy higher education systems worldwide are similar in course length, most are approximately 5-6 years if pre-entry standards and internships are included. The Bachelor of Pharmacy (BPharm) is the most common undergraduate academic degree in the field of pharmacy, being a prerequisite for registration to practice as a pharmacist. However, in the last years, a transition to the clinically orientated Doctor of Pharmacy (PharmD) degree in many countries was seen to be a means of further developing the profession.

Compared to the BPharm, the PharmD curriculum was extended by around one year to include additional pharmacotherapy and patient care coursework, and to expand experiential learning with specified activities towards clinical skills (e.g. patient's counseling, advising other healthcare professionals on drug use issues) (Supapaan, Low, Wongpoowarak, Moolasarn, & Anderson, 2019).

The United States of America was the first country that has moved to a 6-year PharmD degree focused on clinical pharmacy, and most schools and colleges offer a program including basics subjects Drug Information courses (Brazeau et al., 2009; Nkansah et al., 2010).

Considering the complexity of the Drug Information field and the expanding roles of pharmacists as information resources, students should be trained thoroughly in the skills necessary for handling information (Walton, 2006; Wright et al., 2014). However, prior to entering pharmacy schools and faculties, many students lack basic library and information research skills, and all need instruction to reach necessary levels of bibliographic and drug information expertise.

Moreover, students should be able to apply theoretical knowledge and research methods to problem-oriented case studies and real-life clinical situations (Beck, 1980; Walton, 2006; Wood, Morrison, & Oppenheimer, 1990). For this to occur, the teaching of curricular units such as Drug Information should be mandatory to provide students an overview of drug information resources, and retrieval and use of evidence.

The Accreditation Council for Pharmacy Education (ACPE) and the Center for the Advancement of Pharmacy Education (CAPE) emphasize a patient-centered care practice and note that the curriculum must produce graduates with mature critical thinking and problem-solving skills, and the ability to self-direct their learning (Pires & Cavaco, 2019).

In the early 2000s, a survey in the United States revealed that in curriculum Drug Information services teaching and training courses were carried out in 84% and 91% of pharmacy schools (n=75), respectively (Davis & Kruck, 1994; Wang, Troutman, Seo, Peak, & Rosenberg, 2006). Attempts to improve these numbers were made in the country.

Educational institutions such as the University of Kentucky, Southern California University, and Norris Medical Library revised the curriculum to integrate Drug Information services skills and contents throughout the curriculum. Training programs for pharmacists such as the Department of Drug information Service at Iowa University were also developed to customize drug information training in individual schedules (e.g. 2-12 weeks) (Wang, et al., 2006).

However, although almost mandatory, the availability of Drug Information courses and training programs in the Pharmacy curricula seems not to be enough for students to achieve learning outcomes. At the University of Tennessee, for instance, the Drug Information and Literature Evaluation course is a 2-hour course of the second-professional year. Traditional drug information, literature evaluation, and drug use policy, taught primarily through didactic lectures every week, account for the majority of the course.

Past examinations have shown that students struggle with some of the educational contents, particularly biomedical literature evaluation topics. Course evaluations have also indicated that students do not understand the application of course material to the pharmacy career or to the practice of pharmacy. This can be due, amongst others, the educational methods used to teach the Drug Information unit (Timpe, Motl, & Eichner, 2006).

Teaching Drug Information

The back-to-basics traditional education method, also known as conventional education, conceptualizes the teacher as the 'centerpiece' of the teaching-learning process. The teachers communicate the knowledge on a certain topic and enforce standards of behavior in order to established customs, while students are required to listen and study materials. In this way, teachers ensure that students are reward for their efforts, use class periods efficiently and exercise clear rules.

Traditional methods rely mainly on textbooks and lectures, emphasizes on basic skills and assessment is seen as a separate activity that occurs through testing. These include as teaching methods: teacher-centric classrooms, chalk talk methods (i.e. monologue presentation) and few or lack of collaboration/group learning (Belia & et al., 2013).

However, nowadays, the technology-driven academic world moved the medical knowledge-flow from the conventional classrooms to modern learning process. The modern way of teaching is more 'active' and aim to create a variety of situations in which students evolve critical thinking.

That is to say, learners possess a unique set of perceptions and expectations, and are the center of the teaching-learning process (learner-centered models). Modern education methods include technology-driven classrooms, cross-curricular connections, continuous comprehensive evaluation, inquiry-based learning, smart interactive boards, collaborative learning, differential learning, activity-based learning, flipped classroom, problem-based learning (Belia & et al., 2013; Pires & Cavaco, 2019).

Classically, students' learning outcomes may be classified into three domains (Pires & Cavaco, 2019), as follows:

1. **Knowledge:** What students know or understand.

2. **Skills:** What students can do or how they apply their knowledge and understanding.
3. **Competencies:** The context in which knowledge and skills can be applied.

The standards in Pharmacy education are constantly changing or being updated (e.g. introduction of competencies in pharmacy degree syllabi, a transition to a clinically orientated degree) and yet, the biggest problem facing teachers today is the lack of ability of most students to think critically. This could be due to the fact that critical thinking was not effectively promoted within the traditional teaching environment which is mostly based on memorization (Azer, et al., 2013).

In this context, special attention is required during the implementation of complex educational units such as Drug Information. A key requirement for the future is the need to prepare students to participate in the information society, where knowledge is the most crucial factor in the social and economic development of a country, including the field of healthcare.

The adoption of new information technologies and communication has led to significant changes in both the structure and the functionality of education. The introduction of new technologies led to the development and dissemination of web-based learning, electronic learning (e-learning), and distance learning courses thereby offering a new dimension to the provision and content of education.

As a consequence, modern education approaches require students to be responsible for learning the course content outside the classroom, while teachers are responsible for guiding students in subsequent practice modules (Pires & Cavaco, 2019).

In this sense, active learning and training methodologies have been progressively implemented to increase problem-solving and critical-thinking skills of students in a more student-centered environment. Examples of active learning instructional strategies include evaluating case studies, video recordings, class discussions, problem-based learning, simulation (role-playing, simulated patient, and virtual patient), game-based learning, and building concept maps.

In this scenario, students have to face real-life situations that will foster learning and knowledge use, being able to apply course materials, engage in active discussion with colleagues, and strengthen their ability and confidence in resolve problems. Besides, the integration of pharmacy students as members of the healthcare team in real clinical settings, such as hospitals or community pharmacies, to develop skills and improving patient health, is a common pedagogic approach (Akdeniz & et al., 2016; Azer, et al., 2013).

Other interesting teaching alternatives to be used in the Drug Information unit are flipped classes, defined as a teaching technique where the customary teaching environment is switched around by delivering instructional material, frequently online, outside of the classroom, and before the actual classroom lecture. These classes may be based on problem sets, quiz games, mini-lectures, debates, mind mapping, calculations, review sessions, and cases or team-based learning (Pires & Cavaco, 2019; Timpe, et al., 2006).

Case-based learning is a teaching strategy that uses a case-based method that lets students participate in the discussion of detailed scenarios that resemble or typically are real-world examples. This technique is learner-focused and can be done individually, in a small group, or as a class. Case-based is more beneficial when it is done with a facilitator to assist the students through the case. Similarly, team-based learning is an organized form of small-group learning that enhances student development out of class and implementation of knowledge in class. Students are structured strategically into different teams (e.g. 5-7 students) that will work together throughout the class.

They are given an assignment to aid discussion of the case study or additional aspects of content. This strategy requires prior preparation and content assimilation through the class by the educator. Both approaches can also benefit from discussion-based learning, an educational method that concentrates on students gaining knowledge and skills through conversation and dialogue rather than non-participative strategies that focus on lectures, reading, or observations. It is typically used with other tactics including case studies (Pires & Cavaco, 2019; Timpe, et al., 2006).

Considering the above-mention on the complexity of Drug Information and its importance as an educational unit for pharmacist students, the teaching-learning process should be a 'mix' of different approaches aiming at improving knowledge acquisition and long-term retention, and clinical skills development. The primary goal of Drug Information as a curricular unit or course should be to familiarize the students with the usefulness and limitations of various sources and types of drug information in different contexts including clinical care, research, and patient healthcare, as well as to develop excellent oral and written skills for drug information retrieval, selection, evaluation, dissemination, and practical use.

Thus, as learning outcomes, at the end of a course on Drug Information, students should be able to: define drug information and drug information sources, identify producers and originators of information as well their benefits and limitations, understand the hierarchy of studies design and evidence level, recommend appropriate drug information sources to meet the needs of each scenario and requestor, demonstrate sufficient skills to apply the concepts of a stepwise approach to retrieve and select drug information for responding to any drug information request, demonstrate familiarity with contemporary drug information retrieval technology, understand the operation of a drug information center and all the main steps to effectively answer a drug information request, appropriately synthesize, oral and written communicate, document and disseminate pertinent drug information to a specific request.

Table 1 summarizes some practical examples of different teaching approaches that can be used in the field of Drug Information courses. Overall, multimodal methods including interactive lectures, student self-learning, and team-based or case-based learning are preferable and present good results.

FUTURE RESEARCH DIRECTIONS

Additional research is needed to determine whether graduates can apply the knowledge and skills learned in the module to the pharmacy practice setting. Additional research is needed to determine whether graduates can apply the knowledge and skills learned in the module to the pharmacy practice setting.

Larger research lines with stronger theory-based and study designs are needed to improve drug information teaching and learning. Additional research is also needed to verify whenever graduates can properly apply the updated knowledge and skills learned in the model of pharmacy practice settings. Since the combination of different teaching methods seems to perform better in this context, further studies evaluating the outcomes are needed.

Research should also focus on deepening understanding of professionals' behaviors and effectiveness of medication information in different healthcare settings, as well as healthcare literacy and the use of electronic sources.

CONCLUSION

Pharmacists are involved with drug information and should be able to properly select resources and keep current on new literature and tools to address a variety of drug information requests.

The provision of accurate in-depth drug information requires the development of drug information skills through both didactic and experiential training programs. Students must acquire and retain knowledge as a fundamental core upon which to build their clinical practice.

The combination of different teaching methods seems to be the most efficient approach in this context.

Table 1. Examples of studies reporting teaching methods for Drug Information courses

Author/Year	Study Design	Conclusion
Earl, 2009 (Earl, 2009)	Experimental classes: US Pharmacy School (n=102)	• Formats of teaching: cooperative learning/group-based learning with jigsaw technique and students' writing independent research. • Students agreed that class discussions were a useful learning experience that instigates critical thinking. • 75% of students were able to use drug information knowledge in other courses.
Phillips, 2012 (Phillips, Gabay, Ficzere, & Ward, 2012)	Students survey: US Pharmacy Schools (n=62)	• Mean credit hours of Drug Information course: 2.7. • Drug Information taught alone (40%) or together with literature evaluation or biostatistics (37%). • Most common curricular position: 1st or 2nd year. • Most common formats of teaching: didactic lecture (92%), small-groups (90%), internet-based (81%). • Technologies to instruct in Drug Information: online course (95%), audience response systems (61%), YouTube (14%).
Radwanski, 2012 (Redwanski, 2012)	Course unit adaptation: US Pharmacy School (n=115)	• Format of teaching: team-based learning was incorporated in the Drug Information course covering tertiary literature. • Students scored better in the unit assessment with the new teaching approach (90.3) compared to previous courses (lectures) (81.4). • Students liked to physically look up answers using the databases provided which resembled real life experience. • Times to set up the technique and adequate physical space for teams to collaborate can be limiting factors.
Sousa, 2013 (de Sousa, de Lima David, & Noblat Lde, 2013)	New course module and training: Brazil (n=121)	• A 5-week module training in Drug Information was developed for pharmacy students. • Formats of teaching: lectures and oral presentations. • 55% of students completed the module. • The module was rated 'excellent' by 37% of students, 'very good' by 30%, satisfactory by 12%. • The most often mentioned area of dissatisfaction (52%) was the performance of computers.
Bisrat, 2018 (Bisrat, Abel, Salome, Michael, & Sade, 2018)	Students survey: US Pharmacy School (n=80)	• Drug information class as a 3-credit hour (1st year). • Authors developed a comprehensive teaching method that incorporates various tools: lecture, small group assignment, review case-study, homework individual/group assignments, flipped class (article reading, video, debates, and quizzes). • The student's overall score for the unit was 4.28 (SD 0.66) out of 5.0 points. Students believed that this type of multimodal approach allowed them to synthesize fundamental knowledge and skills.
Sando, 2018 (Sando & Feng, 2018)	Course unit adaptation: US Pharmacy School (n=236)	• Format of teaching: online space-education game to study the top 200 drug information (1st year). • Multiple-choice questions are sent via email every 2 days. After the semester, an examination was performed. • High level of student engagement with the game (>80%). • The rate of correctly answered questions improved by 12%. • Students' self-efficacy to recognize brand/generic names and common indications significantly improved.

REFERENCES

Akdeniz, C. (2016). *Learning and Teaching: Theories, Approaches and Models* (2nd ed.). Çözüm Eğitim Yayıncılık.

ALA Presidential Committee on Information Literacy. (1989). *Final Report: American Library Association*. Author.

AlHaqwi, A. I., Kuntze, J., & van der Molen, H. T. (2014). Development of the clinical learning evaluation questionnaire for undergraduate clinical education: Factor structure, validity, and reliability study. *BMC Medical Education*, *14*(1), 44. doi:10.1186/1472-6920-14-44 PMID:24592913

Alper, B. S., Hand, J. A., Elliott, S. G., Kinkade, S., Hauan, M. J., Onion, D. K., & Sklar, B. M. (2004). How much effort is needed to keep up with the literature relevant for primary care? *Journal of the Medical Library Association: JMLA*, *92*(4), 429–437. PMID:15494758

American Pharmacists Association. (2007). *Drug Information Handbook* (15th ed.). Lexi-Comp Inc.

Amerson, A. B., & Wallingford, D. M. (1983). Twenty years' experience with drug information centers. *American Journal of Hospital Pharmacy*, *40*(7), 1172–1178. doi:10.1093/ajhp/40.7.1172 PMID:6881155

Amundstuen Reppe, L., Spigset, O., & Schjott, J. (2016). Drug Information Services Today: Current Role and Future Perspectives in Rational Drug Therapy. *Clinical Therapeutics*, *38*(2), 414–421. doi:10.1016/j.clinthera.2015.12.019 PMID:26831829

Augustin, M. (2014). How to learn effectively in medical school: Test yourself, learn actively, and repeat in intervals. *The Yale Journal of Biology and Medicine*, *87*(2), 207–212. PMID:24910566

Azer, S. A., Guerrero, A. P., & Walsh, A. (2013). Enhancing learning approaches: Practical tips for students and teachers. *Medical Teacher*, *35*(6), 433–443. doi:10.3109/0142159X.2013.775413 PMID:23496121

Badyal, D. K., & Singh, T. (2017). Learning Theories: The Basics to Learn in Medical Education. *International Journal of Applied & Basic Medical Research*, *7*(5, Suppl 1), S1–S3. doi:10.4103/ijabmr.IJABMR_385_17 PMID:29344448

Bansback, N., Keystone, E., O'Dell, J., Phibbs, C. S., Hannagan, K., Brophy, M., & Anis, A. (2015). Making smart investment decisions in clinical research. *Trials*, *16*(1), 590. doi:10.118613063-015-1123-1 PMID:26712327

Beck, R. J. (1980). Drug information program builds skills. *American Pharmacy*, *NS20*(1), 54. doi:10.1016/S0160-3450(15)32924-X PMID:7369124

Belia, D. (2013). Traditional Teaching Methods Vs. Teaching Through The Application Of Information And Communication Technologies In The Accounting Field: Quo Vadis? *European Scientific Journal*, *9*(28).

Berland, G. K., Elliott, M. N., Morales, L. S., Algazy, J. I., Kravitz, R. L., Broder, M. S., Kanouse, D. E., Muñoz, J. A., Puyol, J.-A., Lara, M., Watkins, K. E., Yang, H., & McGlynn, E. A. (2001). Health information on the Internet: Accessibility, quality, and readability in English and Spanish. *Journal of the American Medical Association*, *285*(20), 2612–2621. doi:10.1001/jama.285.20.2612 PMID:11368735

Bernknopf, A. C., Karpinski, J. P., McKeever, A. L., Peak, A. S., Smith, K. M., Smith, W. D., Timpe, E. M., & Ward, K. E. (2009). Drug information: From education to practice. *Pharmacotherapy*, *29*(3), 331–346. doi:10.1592/phco.29.3.331 PMID:19249951

Bisrat, H., Abel, B., Salome, W., Michael, M., & Sade, H. (2018). Development of a New Innovative Teaching Method Using a Comprehensive Approach: A Survey of Students' Opinion. *Biomedical Journal of Scientific & Technical Research*, *3*(4).

Brazeau, G. A., Meyer, S. M., Belsey, M., Bednarczyk, E. M., Bilic, S., Bullock, J., DeLander, G. E., Fiese, E. F., Giroux, S. L., McNatty, D., Nemire, R., Prescott, W. A. Jr, & Traynor, A. P. (2009). Preparing pharmacy graduates for traditional and emerging career opportunities. *American Journal of Pharmaceutical Education*, *73*(8), 157. doi:10.5688/aj7308157 PMID:20221350

Broadwell, M. (1969). *Teaching for learning (XVI)*. The Gospel Guardian.

Carvalho, P. F., & Goldstone, R. L. (2015). The benefits of interleaved and blocked study: Different tasks benefit from different schedules of study. *Psychonomic Bulletin & Review*, *22*(1), 281–288. doi:10.375813423-014-0676-4 PMID:24984923

Chapman, D. (2009). Advanced search features of PubMed. *Journal of the Canadian Academy of Child and Adolescent Psychiatry*, *18*(1), 58–59. PMID:19270851

Chequeta, A., & Lewis, C. (2009). *How Providers Can Lower Costs and Improve Patient Care Using Evidence Based Medicine*. Oracle Corporation.

Clauson, K. A., Marsh, W. A., Polen, H. H., Seamon, M. J., & Ortiz, B. I. (2007). Clinical decision support tools: Analysis of online drug information databases. *BMC Medical Informatics and Decision Making*, *7*(1), 7. doi:10.1186/1472-6947-7-7 PMID:17346336

Cummings, M. (1967). The role of the National Library of Medicine in the national biomedical library network. *Annals of the New York Academy of Sciences*, *142*(2), 503–512. doi:10.1111/j.1749-6632.1967.tb14365.x PMID:5230953

Davies, K., & Harrison, J. (2007). The information-seeking behaviour of doctors: A review of the evidence. *Health Information and Libraries Journal*, *24*(2), 78–94. doi:10.1111/j.1471-1842.2007.00713.x PMID:17584211

Davis, S., & Kruck, L. (1994). Drug information training and experience at U.S. schools of pharmacy. *American Journal of Pharmaceutical Education*, *58*(2).

de Sousa, I. C., de Lima David, J. P., & Noblat Lde, A. (2013). A drug information center module to train pharmacy students in evidence-based practice. *American Journal of Pharmaceutical Education*, *77*(4), 80. doi:10.5688/ajpe77480 PMID:23716748

Dee, C. (2007). The development of the Medical Literature Analysis and Retrieval System (MEDLARS). *Journal of the Medical Library Association: JMLA*, *95*(4), 416–425. doi:10.3163/1536-5050.95.4.416 PMID:17971889

Dee, C. R. (2007). The development of the Medical Literature Analysis and Retrieval System (MEDLARS). *Journal of the Medical Library Association: JMLA*, *95*(4), 416–425. doi:10.3163/1536-5050.95.4.416 PMID:17971889

Delwiche, F. A. (2008). Searching MEDLINE via PubMed. *Clinical Laboratory Science*, *21*(1), 35–41. PMID:18335860

Dickinson, R., Raynor, D. K., Knapp, P., & MacDonald, J. (2017). How much information about the benefits of medicines is included in patient leaflets in the European Union? - A survey. *International Journal of Pharmacy Practice*, *25*(2), 147–158. doi:10.1111/ijpp.12285 PMID:27405658

Drews, J. (2000). Drug discovery: A historical perspective. *Science*, *287*(5460), 1960–1964. doi:10.1126cience.287.5460.1960 PMID:10720314

Earl, G. L. (2009). Using cooperative learning for a drug information assignment. *American Journal of Pharmaceutical Education*, *73*(7), 132. doi:10.5688/aj7307132 PMID:19960089

Eisenberg, M. (2008). Information Literacy: Essential Skills for the Information Age. *DESIDOC Journal of Library and Information Technology*, *28*(2), 39–47. doi:10.14429/djlit.28.2.166

Eysenbach, G., Powell, J., Kuss, O., & Sa, E. R. (2002). Empirical studies assessing the quality of health information for consumers on the world wide web: A systematic review. *Journal of the American Medical Association*, *287*(20), 2691–2700. doi:10.1001/jama.287.20.2691 PMID:12020305

Fischer, J. M. (1980). Modification of the systematic approach to answering drug information requests. *American Journal of Hospital Pharmacy*, *37*(4), 470–476, 472, 476. doi:10.1093/ajhp/37.4.470 PMID:7377208

Ghaibi, S., Ipema, H., & Gabay, M. (2015). ASHP Guidelines on the Pharmacist's Role in Providing Drug Information. *American Journal of Health-System Pharmacy*, *72*(7), 573–577. doi:10.2146p150002 PMID:25788512

Ghaibi, S., Ipema, H., & Gabay, M. (2015). ASHP guidelines on the pharmacist's role in providing drug information. *American Journal of Health-System Pharmacy*, *72*(7), 573–577. doi:10.2146p150002 PMID:25788512

Gonzalez, J., Bryant, S., Hogan, M., Bai, S., Fierro, L., & Hermes-DeSantis, E. R. (2019). Comparison of Postdoctoral Pharmacy Training Programs: Drug Information Residencies and Medical Information Fellowships. *Therapeutic Innovation & Regulatory Science*, *53*(4), 446–454. doi:10.1177/2168479018793375 PMID:30176737

Gonzalez-Gonzalez, A. I., Dawes, M., Sanchez-Mateos, J., Riesgo-Fuertes, R., Escortell-Mayor, E., Sanz-Cuesta, T., & Hernandez-Fernandez, T. (2007). Information needs and information-seeking behavior of primary care physicians. *Annals of Family Medicine*, *5*(4), 345–352. doi:10.1370/afm.681 PMID:17664501

Hersh, W. R., Gorman, P. N., Biagioli, F. E., Mohan, V., Gold, J. A., & Mejicano, G. C. (2014). Beyond information retrieval and electronic health record use: Competencies in clinical informatics for medical education. *Advances in Medical Education and Practice*, *5*, 205–212. doi:10.2147/AMEP.S63903 PMID:25057246

Iwanowicz, S. L., Marciniak, M. W., & Zeolla, M. M. (2006). Obtaining and providing health information in the community pharmacy setting. *American Journal of Pharmaceutical Education*, *70*(3), 57. doi:10.5688/aj700357 PMID:17136178

Kier, K., & Goldwire, M. (2018). Drug Information Resources and Literature Retrieval (7th ed.). ACCP's Pharmacotherapy Self-Assessment Program.

Kruger, J., & Dunning, D. (1999). Unskilled and unaware of it: How difficulties in recognizing one's own incompetence lead to inflated self-assessments. *Journal of Personality and Social Psychology*, *77*(6), 1121–1134. doi:10.1037/0022-3514.77.6.1121 PMID:10626367

Leppink, J., & van den Heuvel, A. (2015). The evolution of cognitive load theory and its application to medical education. *Perspectives on Medical Education*, *4*(3), 119–127. doi:10.100740037-015-0192-x PMID:26016429

Lindberg, D. (2000). Internet access to the National Library of Medicine. Effective clinical practice. *ECP*, *3*(5), 256–260. PMID:11185333

Malone, P., Kier, K., Stanovich, J. E., & Malone, M. J. (2014). *Drug Information: A Guide for Pharmacists* (5th ed.). McGraw-Hill Education.

Manasse, H. R. Jr. (2005). ASHP s 2015 initiative: A collective effort to improve pharmacy practice in hospitals and health-systems in the United States. *Farmacia Hospitalaria*, *29*(6), 349–350. doi:10.1016/S1130-6343(05)73693-X PMID:16433564

Mears, G. (2009). Avoid information overload. Now that you have data, What do you do with it? *JEMS: A Journal of Emergency Medical Services*, *34*(8), 12–15. PMID:19718851

Merigo, J. M., & Nunez, A. (2016). Influential journals in health research: A bibliometric study. *Globalization and Health*, *12*(1), 46. doi:10.118612992-016-0186-4 PMID:27550071

Miranda, G. F., Vercellesi, L., & Bruno, F. (2004). Information sources in biomedical science and medical journalism: Methodological approaches and assessment. *Pharmacological Research*, *50*(3), 267–272. doi:10.1016/j.phrs.2003.12.021 PMID:15225669

Mononen, N., Jarvinen, R., Hameen-Anttila, K., Airaksinen, M., Bonhomme, C., Kleme, J., & Pohjanoksa-Mantyla, M. (2018). A national approach to medicines information research: A systematic review. *Research in Social & Administrative Pharmacy*, *14*(12), 1106–1124. Advance online publication. doi:10.1016/j.sapharm.2018.01.011 PMID:29483046

Nathan, J. P. (2013). Drug information—the systematic approach: Continuing education article. *Journal of Pharmacy Practice*, *26*(2), 78–84. doi:10.1177/0897190012474229 PMID:23519502

National Library of Medicine. (2019). *MeSH (Medical Subject Headings)*. https://www.ncbi.nlm.nih.gov/mesh

Nkansah, N., Mostovetsky, O., Yu, C., Chheng, T., Beney, J., Bond, C. M., & Bero, L. (2010). Effect of outpatient pharmacists' non-dispensing roles on patient outcomes and prescribing patterns. *Cochrane Database of Systematic Reviews*, (7), CD000336. doi:10.1002/14651858.CD000336.pub2 PMID:20614422

Oberauer, K., & Lewandowsky, S. (2008). Forgetting in immediate serial recall: Decay, temporal distinctiveness, or interference? *Psychological Review*, *115*(3), 544–576. doi:10.1037/0033-295X.115.3.544 PMID:18729591

Pennycook, G., Ross, R. M., Koehler, D. J., & Fugelsang, J. A. (2017). Dunning-Kruger effects in reasoning: Theoretical implications of the failure to recognize incompetence. *Psychonomic Bulletin & Review*, *24*(6), 1774–1784. doi:10.375813423-017-1242-7 PMID:28224482

Phillips, J. A., Gabay, M. P., Ficzere, C., & Ward, K. E. (2012). Curriculum and instructional methods for drug information, literature evaluation, and biostatistics: Survey of US pharmacy schools. *The Annals of Pharmacotherapy*, *46*(6), 793–801. doi:10.1345/aph.1Q813 PMID:22669797

Pires, C., & Cavaco, A. (2019). Scoping Pharmacy Students' Learning Outcomes: Where Do We Stand? *Pharmacy (Basel, Switzerland)*, *7*(1), 23. Advance online publication. doi:10.3390/pharmacy7010023 PMID:30818854

Redwanski, J. (2012). Incorporating Team-Based Learning in a Drug Information Course Covering Tertiary Literature. *Currents in Pharmacy Teaching & Learning*, *4*(3), 202–206. doi:10.1016/j.cptl.2012.04.004

Rosenberg, J. M., Koumis, T., Nathan, J. P., Cicero, L. A., & McGuire, H. (2004). Current status of pharmacist-operated drug information centers in the United States. *American Journal of Health-System Pharmacy*, *61*(19), 2023–2032. doi:10.1093/ajhp/61.19.2023 PMID:15509125

Sando, K. R., & Feng, X. (2018). Use of an Online Spaced-Education Game to Study Top 200 Drugs in a Skills Laboratory Course. *American Journal of Pharmaceutical Education*, *82*(7), 6324. doi:10.5688/ajpe6324 PMID:30323387

Schumacher, D. J., Englander, R., & Carraccio, C. (2013). Developing the master learner: Applying learning theory to the learner, the teacher, and the learning environment. *Academic Medicine*, *88*(11), 1635–1645. doi:10.1097/ACM.0b013e3182a6e8f8 PMID:24072107

Sharma, N. (2016). Cognitive load theory and teaching in primary care. *The British Journal of General Practice*, *66*(649), 430. doi:10.3399/bjgp16X686389 PMID:27481975

Sharp, M., Bodenreider, O., & Wacholder, N. (2008). A framework for characterizing drug information sources. *AMIA ... Annual Symposium Proceedings - AMIA Symposium. AMIA Symposium*, 662–666. PMID:18999182

Stansfield, C., Brunton, G., & Rees, R. (2014). Search wide, dig deep: Literature searching for qualitative research. An analysis of the publication formats and information sources used for four systematic reviews in public health. *Research Synthesis Methods*, *5*(2), 142–151. doi:10.1002/jrsm.1100 PMID:26052653

Supapaan, T., Low, B. Y., Wongpoowarak, P., Moolasarn, S., & Anderson, C. (2019). A transition from the BPharm to the PharmD degree in five selected countries. *Pharmacy Practice*, *17*(3), 1611. doi:10.18549/PharmPract.2019.3.1611 PMID:31592299

Taine, S. I. (1963). The Medical Literature Analysis and Retrieval System. *Bulletin of the Medical Library Association*, *51*, 157–167. PMID:13980229

Thiele, R., Poiro, N., Scalzo, D., & Nemergut, E. (2010). Speed, accuracy, and confidence in Google, Ovid, PubMed, and UpToDate: Results of a randomized trial. *Postgraduate Medical Journal*, *86*(1018), 459–465. doi:10.1136/pgmj.2010.098053 PMID:20709767

Tietze, K. J. (2012). *Researching and Providing Drug Information Clinical Skills for Pharmacists* (3rd ed.). Mosby.

Timpe, E. M., Motl, S. E., & Eichner, S. F. (2006). Weekly active-learning activities in a drug information and literature evaluation course. *American Journal of Pharmaceutical Education*, *70*(3), 52. doi:10.5688/aj700352 PMID:17136173

Walton, C. A. (2006). Education and training of the drug information specialist. 1967. *The Annals of Pharmacotherapy*, *40*(2), 311–315. doi:10.1345/aph.140008 PMID:16452084

Wang, F., Troutman, W. G., Seo, T., Peak, A., & Rosenberg, J. M. (2006). Drug information education in doctor of pharmacy programs. *American Journal of Pharmaceutical Education*, *70*(3), 51. doi:10.5688/aj700351 PMID:17136172

Watanabe, A. S., McCart, G., Shimomura, S., & Kayser, S. (1975). Systematic approach to drug information requests. *American Journal of Hospital Pharmacy*, *32*(12), 1282–1285. PMID:1211401

Wood, E. H., Morrison, J. L., & Oppenheimer, P. R. (1990). Drug information skills for pharmacy students: Curriculum integration. *Bulletin of the Medical Library Association*, *78*(1), 8–14. PMID:2295022

World Health Organization (WHO). (1996). *Good pharmacy practice (GPP) in community and hospital pharmacy settings* [WHO/PHARM/DAP/96.1]. WHO.

World Health Organization (WHO). (1997). The role of the pharmacist in the health care system, preparing the future pharmacist: curricular development: report of a third WHO Consultative Group on the Role of the Pharmacist. World Health Organization.

Wright, E. A., Brown, B., Gettig, J., Martello, J. L., McClendon, K. S., Smith, K. M., Teeters, J., Ulbrich, T. R., Wegrzyn, N., & Bradley-Baker, L. R. (2014). Teaching and learning curriculum programs: Recommendations for postgraduate pharmacy experiences in education. *American Journal of Health-System Pharmacy, 71*(15), 1292–1302. doi:10.2146/ajhp130657 PMID:25027537

KEY TERMS AND DEFINITIONS

Drug Information: Defined as the discovery, use, and management of information in the use of medications.

Drug Information Center: An operational unit that provide technical and scientific information about drugs in an objective and timely manner.

Drug Information Specialist: The professional (i.e. pharmacist) that has enough expertise and knowledge to retrieve, select, evaluate and disseminate information towards a specific drug-related question.

Information Literacy: Is the ability to recognize when information is needed, then to locate, evaluate the appropriate information, and use it effectively and responsibly.

Information Resource: An infrastructure or material that provides content (data) and information services for the user.

Learning Method: The sequence or conditional learning path of the given learning steps, allowing sequencing, conditions and repetitions of some learning activities.

Literature Search: A systematic and comprehensive search of data, that can be carry out in any available source.

MeSH Terms: Medical Subject Headings is a comprehensive controlled vocabulary for the purpose of indexing journal articles and books in the life sciences at MEDLINE.

Teaching Methods: Comprises the different principles and methods used by teachers to enable student learning.

Chapter 4
Challenges in Evidence-Based Practice Education:
From Teaching Concepts Towards Decision-Making Learning

Helena H. Borba
Department of Pharmacy, Federal University of Paraná, Brazil

Fernanda S. Tonin
Pharmaceutical Sciences Program, Federal University of Paraná, Brazil

Roberto Pontarolo
Department of Pharmacy, Federal University of Paraná, Brazil

Fernando Fernandez-Llimos
Faculty of Pharmacy, University of Porto, Portugal

ABSTRACT

Evidence-based practice is a key element and indicator of high-quality patient care. Healthcare professionals must effectively acquire the necessary knowledge, skills, and attitudes to gather, assess, and interpret the best available evidence in order to ground their clinical decisions. Both achieving competency and delivering instruction in evidence-based practice are complex processes requiring a multimodal approach that may include traditional lectures, interactive teaching strategies, clinically-integrated teaching strategies, active learning. This chapter will provide a brief overview of the concepts of evidence-based practice, interpretation of systematic reviews and meta-analyses, grading evidence, and recommendations' strength. For each topic, teaching strategies or methods will be discussed.

DOI: 10.4018/978-1-7998-4486-0.ch004

INTRODUCTION

Evidence-Based Practice Concepts and Barriers to Its Application in Clinical Practice

Evidence-based practice (EBP) is defined as the thorough use of the best available clinical evidence, aligned with the individual clinical expertise and patients' values and choices, to guide decision-making in the healthcare field (Sackett, Rosenberg, Gray, Haynes, & Richardson, 1996).

Critical thinking is a key element for EBP, whose practice can be summarized into five crucial steps:

Step 1: Formulate an answerable research question-based on the healthcare professional needs
Step 2: Detect the best evidence for answering the research question
Step 3: Critically assess the retrieved evidence and its value
Step 4: Apply the findings into clinical practice / decision-making
Step 5: Assess the performance

The development of these competences is crucial for practicing healthcare professionals to provide high-quality healthcare. Hence, it is necessary to effectively implement EBP in healthcare professionals' curricula (Hung et al., 2019; Larsen, Terkelsen, Carlsen, & Kristensen, 2019; Young, Rohwer, Volmink, & Clarke, 2014).

Despite the positive attitude of healthcare professionals towards EBP for improving patient outcomes, several studies pointed to the little use of the evidence to guide their practice. For instance, literature shows that 66% of nurses only read health literature when needed, while around 27% of these professionals often use research findings in practice. Additionally, it is estimated that only one in four healthcare professionals incorporates EBP to guide decision-making in health settings (Andiwatir & Betan, 2019; Patelarou et al., 2017).

Once the number of EBP practitioners is increasing, it is assumed that evidence-based practice is a learnable competence. Nevertheless, significant barriers have been reported by healthcare professionals, specifically nurses, for not engaging in EBP. These barriers include lack of time, resources, and knowledge, difficulties in assessing research, and lack of perception of the benefits of applying EBP into clinical practice.

Moreover, most of the health students are taught only the first three steps of EBP, lacking the knowledge to perform the last two steps in clinical practice, which is, integrating evidence into clinical decision-making and evaluating changes in patients' outcomes. In this sense, the most appropriate methods for teaching EBP in undergraduate, postgraduate, and continuing medical education programs have been explored over the years (Hatala & Guyatt, 2002; Horntvedt, Nordsteien, Fermann, & Severinsson, 2018; Larsen et al., 2019; Long et al., 2016).

Evidence-Based Practice Teaching Methods Framework

In order to evaluate the best teaching approach, it is important to assess learning achievement, which includes knowledge, skills, attitudes and behavior. The first one refers to defining and understanding the meaning of concepts, which can be applied to given problems and be translated into developed skills. Changes in attitudes are observed when one recognizes the need of employing a certain knowledge or skill in practice. At last, when one looks for the available evidence and uses the knowledge and skills to guide clinical practice, a change in the behavior is noticed. The sustained changes in the clinicians' behavior are expected to promote improvements in patients' health outcomes (Khan & Coomarasamy, 2006).

The existing teaching methods can be didactic, interactive, or mixed, including workshops, journal clubs, lectures, which can be integrated with clinical practice. Moreover, the teaching approach can involve face-to-face contact, online sessions, or a mixed strategy (Khan & Coomarasamy, 2006; Young et al., 2014).

Khan and Coomarasamy (2006) developed a hierarchy of effective teaching and learning skills, professional attitudes and behaviors on EBP for healthcare professionals. At the bottom, lies the didactic, classroom or standalone teaching activities, which will unlikely improve clinicians' competences or patient's health outcomes due to the lack of interactivity inherent to this teaching method and the consequent superficial learning. Above, there is the interactive classroom-based teaching or the didactic clinically integrated teaching. The interactive and integrated approaches ease the perception of the relevance and application of EBP knowledge in the clinical practice, which favors the learning process. At the top of the hierarchy lie the interactive and clinically integrated teaching activities, representing the most effective method for teaching EBP. This approach promotes deeper learning, since information is directly relevant to clinical practice, facilitating students' learning (Horntvedt et al., 2018; Khan & Coomarasamy, 2006).

In 2016, Kyriakoulis et al. (2016) published a systematic review assessing educational strategies to teach EBP to undergraduate health students. Of the 20 included studies, 17 have been published after 2010, demonstrating how recent the investigations over the topic are. The methods to teach EBP included tutorials, lectures, conferences, online sessions, journal clubs and workshops, with a wide range of duration (from two hours to one year). The main outcomes evaluated in the included studies were knowledge, attitudes, and EBP skills, mostly assessed shortly after the intervention. Overall, the included studies exhibited positive results regarding improvements in students' EBP knowledge and skills after the teaching interventions delivery, regardless of the duration of the intervention. Nevertheless, robust evidence on the most effective method to teach EBP to undergraduate health students is still sparse, particularly concerning when introducing EBP into the curriculum (Kyriakoulis et al., 2016).

Effectiveness of Teaching Approaches to Evidence-Based Practice

Despite the availability of different teaching approaches, traditional lectures are still the pillar of the majority of healthcare education programs. The great advantage of this teaching method is that it allows transmitting a wide variety of information. Nevertheless, it is a teaching-centered method, so students assume a passive role, impairing critical thinking and promoting the acquisition of inert knowledge, which hardly can be applied in a real-life setting. Hence, lectures alone are considered the less effective teaching strategy for professional practice disciplines, such as EBP, trapping learners in a disempowering education (Alt, 2015; Applin, Williams, Day, & Buro, 2011).

To overcome the problems of teaching-centered methods, problem-based learning (PBL) has been arising as a notable strategy for healthcare students, since it stimulates learner engagement in the learning process (Applin et al., 2011). PBL is a student-centered teaching method in which learners are aroused to develop problem-solving skills while acquiring knowledge in self-directed learning (Alt, 2015). Through this strategy, students can be encouraged to formulate research questions of their interest, build a search strategy, and perform a systematic search in electronic databases.

BACKGROUND

The literature suggests that environments where the student is an active participant, such as in PBL courses, favor the learning process because the learner engages in reflection and acquires experience. Therefore, a constructivist approach leads to transformative learning (Horntvedt et al., 2018). The constructivist philosophy embraces the perception of the learner as an active and responsible agent in the process of knowledge acquisition.

Hereupon, constructivist practices may enhance learning self-efficacy (i.e. individual beliefs in its own competence to successfully acting to achieve an academic goal), which is a meaningful psychological construct in the context of learning. Academic self-efficacy is associated with students' persistence and motivation in developing skills and attitudes (Alt, 2015). In this sense, it is important to consider that the level of confidence with attitudes prior to graduation highly influences the intention to use EBP in future clinical practice (Ramis et al., 2019).

A constructivist learning environment includes key features, beginning with the recognition that learning is an active process and that knowledge is not certain. Since learning is also a social activity, the process should stimulate interaction and collaboration among learners. Materials and resources, when used, should be individualized according to students' needs, and meta-cognitive (i.e. *the act of thinking about thinking* (Flavell, 1979)) strategies should be encouraged, as the critical and reflective thinking.

Finally, the learning process should be grounded in contextually significant settings (Alt, 2015). It is theorized that meta-cognition is among the strongest predictors of learning, once an effective learning process requires the individual to recognize what he knows and what he does not know, as well as what helps him to learn (Langdon et al., 2019).

Evidence has shown that offering flexible studying methods, such as online material, which enables learning outside the campus, favors students' engagement and knowledge attainment, consisting of a more effective teaching strategy than the traditional lecture. Additionally, the use of e-learning technology eases the interaction between education and practice and facilitates the involvement of educators in student teaching (Mary, Julie, & Jennifer, 2014).

To overcome some barriers to EBP engaging, a web-based, evidence-based research tool, which can be accessed by healthcare professionals from a computer or smartphone, was developed. The main goal of such a tool was to guide students in detecting and critically appraising the available scientific literature, retrieved from quality electronic databases, avoiding that healthcare professionals rely on personal experience only to make clinical decisions.

Data from the preliminary study evaluating the effectiveness of the tool indicates that it enhanced overall EBP skills so that the tool enriches the list of available teaching methods supporting evidence-based practice (Long et al., 2016). These findings are in accordance with the results from the scoping review conducted by Larsen et al., in which the use of information technology was pointed to be mainly positive for undergraduate healthcare students in the context of EBP teaching (Larsen et al., 2019).

In a systematic review, Khan and Coomarasamy (2006) showed that teaching EBP integrated into clinical practice, rather than adopting a classroom teaching approach, promotes positive changes in attitudes and behaviors in post-graduates. Larsen et al. (2019). in a scoping review assessing methods for teaching EBP for undergraduate healthcare students, identified that collaboration with clinical practice is a key strategy in the context of effective EBP learning.

Integrating EBP concepts to the clinical practicum has proven to be the most effective teaching strategy, decreasing barriers and empowering students' application of EBP in practice (Andiwatir & Betan, 2019; Horntvedt et al., 2018). Moreover, theory-based interventions should be contemplated considering that effective EBP learning comprises cognitive, affective, behavioral and environmental components (Khan & Coomarasamy, 2006).

Fernandez et al. (2014) compared four teaching strategies on EBP skills among postgraduate nursing students: standard distance teaching method; computer laboratory teaching method, in which students received feedback on their work during the practical training workshop; EBP-DVD teaching method, which simulated the computer laboratory teaching method and incorporated self-learning; and didactic classroom teaching method, in which students received face-to-face lectures during the teaching semester. The authors found that the EBP-DVD teaching method was superior to the other approaches in providing the students with EBP skills. It was postulated that this strategy demands the active engagement of students in the learning process, which is essential for competence development on EBP. The DVD enables the student to review the content of the class multiple times, which makes this method an effective teaching approach for postgraduate nursing students (Khan & Coomarasamy, 2006).

Data from systematic reviews indicate that a multifaceted approach (i.e. a combination of teaching strategies including lectures, group discussions, journal clubs, and computer lab sessions), given over a few weeks, are more effective than single interventions presented over a short duration in improving EBP competence amongst undergraduates, residents and practicing health professionals (Kyriakoulis et al., 2016; Young et al., 2014).

Embed librarians to support students in managing evidence search procedures and assist them to critically appraise the retrieved information, is also an effective strategy explored in a few studies. As librarians are experts in the EBP field, they may help students to develop information literacy skills (Larsen et al., 2019). Furthermore, the use of online material and information technologies, through simulation, mobile devices, electronic health records, clinical decision support systems, may facilitate EBP teaching (Long et al., 2016). E-learning technologies in educational activities have the advantage of not being limited by time or spot, such as lectures, which facilitate information access and its application by students in clinical practice (Khan & Coomarasamy, 2006).

Despite the greater effectiveness of integrated teaching methods, in which students can experience the application of EBP in clinical settings, translating evidence into practice is not an easy task. Hence, simulation-based teaching may be a suitable approach to overcome barriers related to practical learning. With this strategy, students are exposed to different simulated patient care scenarios, which stimulates critical thinking and problem-solving. This approach, therefore, arouses EBP competences development as well as its application into clinical practice, promoting optimal patient care (Hung et al., 2019).

It is important to notice that learners have different learning styles, therefore requiring a range of teaching methods (Applin et al., 2011). To enable the development of competencies in EBP, students and healthcare professionals should have a background in epidemiology, biostatistics, electronic databases search, and critical inquiry philosophy (Young et al., 2014). Therefore, it was suggested by nursing scholars that EBP teaching should be introduced in the undergraduate nursing curriculum, integrating EBP concepts throughout the course, in order to fulfill the future practice needs of these healthcare professionals (Hung et al., 2019). Literature supports that EBP courses should be delivered early in the curriculum of healthcare students, once the early introduction of this subject has shown to produce high levels of satisfaction from the students in addition to success in this field (Mary et al., 2014).

Effective EBP teaching strategies also improve analytical skills, as shown by a few studies evaluating nursing students. These skills may change attitudes concerning the use of research in clinical practice, improving clinical judgment, and positively reflecting on patient outcomes (Horntvedt et al., 2018).

In summary, regardless of the teaching strategy, encouraging EBP learning among academics and healthcare professionals is undeniably associated with improvements in clinical practice delivery. Concerning the teaching method, interactive approaches, such as online group discussions, enable personalized feedback and encourages interaction between educator and student, which favors adult learning (Patelarou et al., 2017).

The following topics of this chapter provide supporting material for EBP learners to ease the grasp on systematic reviews, meta-analysis, grading evidence and recommendations' strength interpretation.

INTERPRETATION OF SYSTEMACTIC REVIEWS AND META-ANALYSES

Considering the hierarchy of evidence, systematic reviews with or without meta-analysis, lie on the top of the hierarchy pyramid, representing the higher level of available evidence. Despite some recent revisions on the evidence pyramid structure, for didactic means, we kept the simplistic design, presented in Figure 1, is recommended (Evans, 2003; Murad, Asi, Alsawas, & Alahdab, 2016)

Figure 1. Evidence hierarchy pyramid
Source: Adapted from Murad, 2016 and Evans, 2003.

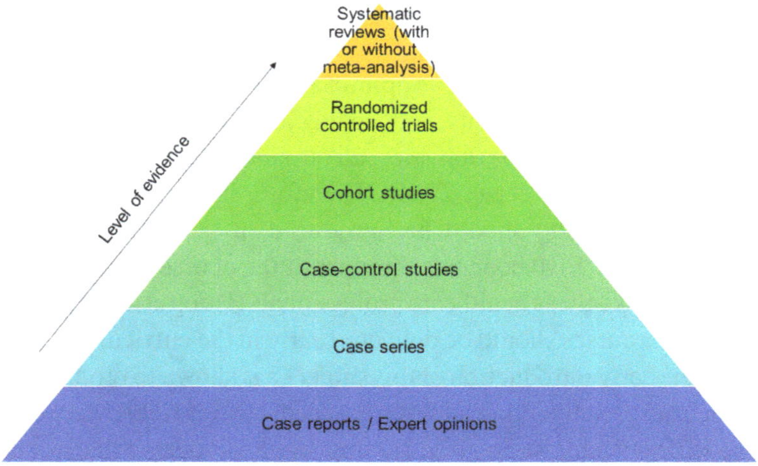

To practice EBP, students and healthcare professionals must know how to conduct and interpret a systematic review. In this sense, guidelines from the Cochrane Collaboration and the Joanna Briggs Institute may help researches in the conduct and interpretation of this type of study. In addition, EBP practitioners and learners should be aware that systematic reviews must follow the Preferred Reporting Items for Systematic Review and Meta-analysis statement (PRISMA checklist 2009) (Aromataris & Munn, 2017; Higgins & Green, 2011 ; Moher et al., 2009).

Properly conducting a systematic review involves the execution of several steps, which will be following depicted (Tawfik et al., 2019).

1. **Formulating a Research Question:** The research question should be feasible, relevant and follow ethical precepts. The PICOS (Population, Intervention, Comparison, Outcome, Study design) tool may be used to help the researcher to formulate a clear and well-defined research question. An example of a research question, following the PICOS tool, could be:

   P - Adult patients with a throat infection
   I - Antibiotic A
   C - Antibiotic B
   O - Efficacy (infection resolution)
   S - Randomized controlled trials

This, the research question could be formulated as "Has antibiotic A demonstrated having a better efficacy profile than antibiotic B in experimental studies for the treatment of adults with throat infection?"

2. **Conducting a Preliminary Search:** This step is important to identify relevant articles, guarantee that the research question was not answered by previous studies and that are enough articles to conduct the proposed systematic review. Using the former example, a simple search in Pubmed, Scopus, or Google Scholar using search terms as "throat infection" AND ("antibiotic A" OR "antibiotic B") AND systematic review could be conducted. If systematic reviews with the same goal were not retrieved and if enough studies addressing the subject of the research question are identified, the research question is feasible and interesting.
3. **Defining Inclusion and Exclusion Criteria:** Inclusion and exclusion criteria should be clearly defined in advance, to avoid any bias in the further steps. PICOS reflects the inclusion criteria (e.g. randomized controlled trials addressing adult patients with a throat infection that were treated with antibiotic A or antibiotic B reporting data on infection resolution will be included). Exclusion criteria should be defined having in mind what should be excluded after applying the inclusion criteria. Examples of exclusion criteria could be articles published in non-Roman characters (e.g. Japanese, Chinese), or studies without a parallel control group.
4. **Elaborating the Search Strategy:** The search strategy is built based on the PICOS, of the formulated research question. Search descriptors should comprise free-text terms, which are included in the titles and abstracts of the articles, as well as index terms (e.g. MeSH [Medical Subject Headings] terms). Additionally, Pubmed offers clinical queries to help researchers to build their search strategies. The search terms should then be combined through Boolean operators, such as AND and OR. An example of a search strategy for Pubmed is presented below. The search should be adapted to each specific electronic database selected by the research team (e.g. Scopus, Web of Science). An example of a search strategy for PubMed could be:

Pharyngitis[MH] OR pharyngitis[TIAB] OR pharyngitides[TIAB] OR "sore throat"[TIAB] OR "sore throats"[TIAB](terms referring to the clinical condition)
AND

*"Antibiotic A"[MH] OR "antibiotic A"[TIAB] OR "Antibiotic B"[MH] OR "antibiotic B"[TIAB](terms referring to the evaluated treatments)***AND**

(clinical[TIAB] AND trial[TIAB]) OR "clinical trials as a topic"[MH] OR "clinical trial"[PT] OR random[TIAB] OR "random allocation"[MH] OR "therapeutic use"[SH] (terms referring to the study design)*

5. **Performing the Search in the Selected Databases and Exporting the Retrieved Articles to a Library and an Excel Sheet:** The AMSTAR guidelines recommend that the searches should be performed in at least two databases (Shea et al., 2017). Examples of medical databases include Pubmed, Scopus, Web of Science, Cochrane Library, Scielo, DOAJ). The articles retrieved through the electronic searches should be exported to a reference manager software (e.g. Endnote) to remove the duplicates, and then exported to a spreadsheet (e.g. Excel) with the essential information (e.g. authors' names, article title, publication year, abstract) to perform the screening phase.
6. **Writing and Registration of a Protocol:** A protocol of the systematic review, including the research question, eligibility criteria, assessed intervention, quality appraisal and analysis plan should be written and submitted to a registry site, as PROSPERO. The protocol registration assures transparency of the systematic review process and is considered a documented proof of the planned work.
7. **Screening the Retrieved Studies by Titles and Abstracts:** To exclude non-relevant references, two independent reviewers should read the titles and abstracts of the articles. An over-inclusive approach should be adopted in this step to avoid the accidental exclusion of relevant studies. At the end of this phase, the two reviewers select, in a consensus, the studies that will be evaluated for inclusion by analysis of their full-text. In cases of disagreements, a third reviewer must be consulted.
8. **Full-Text Appraisal:** To exclude references based on the pre-specified eligibility criteria, the studies not excluded in the screening phase should be downloaded and fully read by two independent reviewers. The reasons for articles' exclusions should be reported to ensure the transparency of the process. In cases of disagreements, a third reviewer must be consulted.
9. **Performing a Manual Search:** To guarantee that all relevant studies were retrieved, and minimize the weaknesses of search strategies and bibliographic databases, an additional manual search is recommended. To perform this step, the reference lists of included articles should be searched to identify possibly relevant reports that may not be recovered by the initial search.
10. **Extracting Data and Assessing Quality:** In this step, the two reviewers, independently, will extract the data from the included articles in an extraction form (e.g. Excel spreadsheet) *ad hoc* created for the study. Relevant extracted information should include the author's names, article title, year of publication,

country, number of patients, patient' age and gender, clinical outcomes of interest (e.g. cure rates, adverse events). The extracted data should be compared by the two reviewers and consensus must be achieved. Once the quality of the selected articles highly influences the quality of the evidence produced by a systematic review, the researcher must assess the methodological quality and risk of potential bias of the included studies (Herner, 2019). There are several tools available to appraise studies' quality according to the study design, as the Risk of Bias (ROB) Cochrane tool for randomized controlled trials (Higgins et al., 2011), the New Castle Ottawa tool for cohort and case-control studies (Wells et al., 2000), ROBINS-I tool for non-randomized controlled trials (Sterne et al., 2016), AMSTAR tool for systematic reviews (Shea et al., 2017), CARE tool for case reports (Kuster, De Tonnac, & Papa, 2019). Quality assessment should be performed by two independent reviewers and further discussed to achieve consensus in the results, in order to correct the expected human error and bias.

11. **Combining and Summarizing the Findings**: The main results of the systematic review may be described through qualitative analysis, in which the researchers can elaborate a clean and structured table with the main findings and conclusions of the included articles. If there are enough comparable data (i.e. studies with the same design, comparing the same intervention, at the same dose and treatment regimen) a quantitative analysis (e.g. pairwise meta-analysis) can be performed.

Considering the previous example of a research question (i.e. "Has antibiotic A demonstrated having a better efficacy profile than antibiotic B in experimental studies for the treatment of adults with throat infection?"), and after thoroughly conduct all the aforementioned steps with a sufficient number of studies providing quantitative homogeneous data, the researcher could proceed (inserting the extracted data in an analytical software (e.g. Review Manager, R, Addis). Table 1 shows the hypothetical data extraction for three RCT (Randomized Control Trial).

Table 1. Hypothetical data extraction sheet

Study, Year Treatment	Study Design	Country	Sample Size	Age Median (Range)	Infection Resolution (n)
Study 1, 2018 - Antibiotic A - Antibiotic B	Double-blind RCT	USA	200 100 100	35 (29-60)	87 65
Study 2, 2019 - Antibiotic A - Antibiotic B	Open-label RCT	Canada	360 180 180	28 (19-50)	165 120
Study 3, 2017 - Antibiotic A - Antibiotic B	Double-blind RCT	Multicentric (USA, Canada, Mexico)	1500 750 750	31 (22-58)	720 572

Figure 2. Extracted data insertion in the meta-analysis software performed in Review Manager 5.3

Comparison: 1 Antibiotic A vs Antibiotic B, Outcome: 1.1 Infection resolution

Study or Subgroup	Antibiotic A		Antibiotic B		Weight	Risk Ratio
	Events	Total	Events	Total		M-H, Random, 95% CI
Study 1, 2018	87	100	65	100	10.5%	1.34 [1.14, 1.57]
Study 2, 2019	165	180	120	180	20.0%	1.38 [1.23, 1.54]
Study 3, 2017	720	750	572	750	69.5%	1.26 [1.21, 1.31]
Total (95% CI)		1030		1030	100.0%	1.29 [1.22, 1.36]
Total events	972		757			
Heterogeneity: Tau² = 0.00; Chi² = 2.52, df = 2 (P = 0.28); I² = 21%						
Test for overall effect: Z = 9.04 (P < 0.00001)						

Figure 3. Forest plot with summary results of the meta-analysis performed in Review Manager 5.3

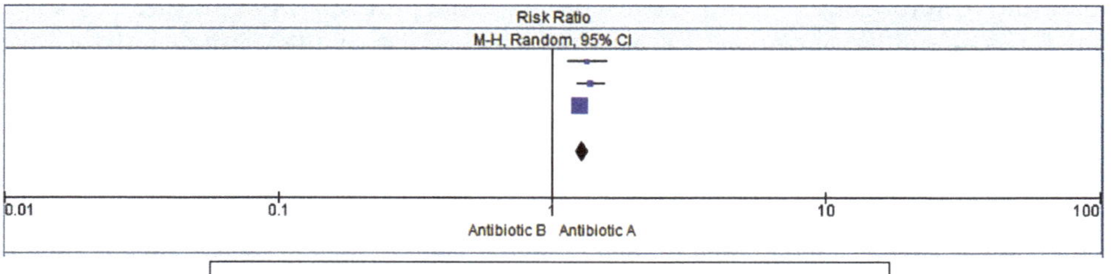

Study or Subgroup	Antibiotic A Events	Antibiotic A Total	Antibiotic B Events	Antibiotic B Total	Weight	Risk Ratio M-H, Random, 95% CI
Study 1, 2018	87	100	65	100	10.5%	1.34 [1.14, 1.57]
Study 2, 2019	165	180	120	180	20.0%	1.38 [1.23, 1.54]
Study 3, 2017	720	750	572	750	69.5%	1.26 [1.21, 1.31]
Total (95% CI)		**1030**		**1030**	**100.0%**	**1.29 [1.22, 1.36]**
Total events	972		757			
Heterogeneity: Tau² = 0.00; Chi² = 2.52, df = 2 (P = 0.28); I² = 21%						
Test for overall effect: Z = 9.04 (P < 0.00001)						

By inserting the extracted data regarding the outcome of interest (infection resolution), as shown in Figure 2, the software will provide the meta-analysis results through a forest-plot (Figure 3).

In this simulated analysis, a forest plot with three studies and their respective risk ratios (RR) followed by the 95% confidence intervals were produced. The blue box represents the effect size (risk ratio, in this example) of each included study.

The size of the blue box indicates the weight of each study in the meta-analysis, which directly correlates to the sample size. The black diamond represents the pooled effect size (in RR) of the three included studies. In this example, the black diamond does not cross the vertical neutrality line (RR = 1), indicating statistically significant difference among the compared groups, favoring the alternative showed on the right side of the plot (Antibiotic A), with a pooled RR of infection resolution of 1.29 (95% CI 1.22 to 1.36). The significant difference is also confirmed by a p-value < 0.05.

The heterogeneity between the included studies can be assessed by the I^2 value ($I^2 = 21\%$). An $I^2 \leq 25\%$ designates low heterogeneity, between 26 and 50% indicates moderate heterogeneity, and above 50% represents a high heterogeneity (Higgins & Green, 2011; Huedo-Medina et al., 2006). In this example, risk ratio as effect measure, the Mantel-Haenszel statistics and a random effect model were used. Nevertheless, the researcher may choose among different statistics according to the analysis and the nature of the assessed variables (dichotomous, or continuous).

Dichotomous variables can be assessed through risk ratio, odds ratio, or risk difference, whereas continuous variables can be evaluated through mean difference or standardized mean difference. Mantel-Haenszel statistics was preferred in the example because it presents good statistical properties when there are few events, which is a common situation when conducting systematic reviews.

Other statistical methods include Peto, indicated for rare events, and the Inverse Variance method, which may produce poor estimates of the standard errors of effect when data are scarce, (i.e. low event rates or small sample sizes. The researcher can also choose to perform the meta-analysis using fixed or random effects model.

When using fixed effects it is assumed that there is no heterogeneity between the included studies, whereas when using random effects model the researcher assumes that heterogeneity is present and the software adjusts the weight of the studies according to the extent of variation. In the complete absence of heterogeneity, both fixed and random effects produce the same result (Cheung & Vijayakumar, 2016; Higgins & Green, 2011).

The accuracy of the results may be evaluated by performing sensitivity analyses, by removing the studies one at a time and observing if the result is significantly modified. In a meta-analysis with high heterogeneity between the included studies, this method is useful to identify if a specific study is responsible for the high levels of I^2.

Once identified, the study should be critically assessed to evaluated and identify the characteristics that may contribute to heterogeneity (e.g. differences in population, such as ethnicity, age, or dissimilarities in the design of the study, such as randomization or blindness of participants). However, no study should be definitely removed from the analysis and the authors of the systematic review should report and discuss the particularities found (Higgins & Green, 2011).

To account for the potential effects of the heterogeneity in the precision of the pooled estimates, the prediction interval should always accompany the confidence interval, and recommendations emerging from the meta-analysis should be considered the significance of the pooled estimate considering the PI (IntHout, Ioannidis, Rovers, & Goeman, 2016).

Grading Evidence and Recommendations' Strength

When performing a systematic review, researchers must assess the confidence that the obtained results are correct, in addition to the confidence that the obtained results may support a specific recommendation, which is translated into the quality of evidence. In this sense, the GRADE (Grading of Recommendations Assessment, Development and Evaluation) system was developed by the GRADE Working Group aiming to provide a structured, transparent and systematic approach for a rating of the evidence.

The use of GRADE by researchers that publish clinical guidelines articles is encouraged by several organizations (e.g. the World Health Organization, the Cochrane Collaboration) and publishers, such as the BMJ, highlighting the relevance of learning how to apply this approach in clinical research and to interpret the results regarding the strength of recommendations (Balshem et al., 2011; G. H. Guyatt, A. D. Oxman, G. E. Vist, et al., 2008).

The GRADE system is applied for each outcome of interest and the researchers should rate the outcome according to its importance to patients and decision making in critical (e.g. mortality), important but not critical (e.g. pain), and not important for decision making or of lower importance to patients (e.g. flatulence). The overall quality of evidence will be determined by the critical outcomes (Gordon H Guyatt et al., 2008).

The assessment of the quality of the evidence by using the GRADE system starts with the study design, assuming that well-conducted randomized controlled trials present high quality, whereas observational studies without exceptional strengths present low-quality evidence. GRADE approach involves five factors that can downgrade the quality of the study, both RCT and observational designs, i.e. limitations, the inconsistency of reports, indirectness of evidence, imprecision and publication bias. On the other hand, some factors can increase the quality of evidence, i.e. a large magnitude of the effect, plausible confounding, and dose-response gradient. After analyzing these elements and applying them to each outcome of interest, the quality of evidence is rated in high, moderate, low, or very low. A summary of how to assess these factors is presented in Table 2 (Gordon H Guyatt et al., 2008).

Table 2. Factors that might decrease or increase the quality of evidence.

Factors That Might Decrease the Quality of Evidence	
Study limitations	Presence of major limitations that may produce bias in the results, e.g. lack of blinding, deficiency in allocation concealment, expressive loss of follow-up.
Inconsistency of reports	Presence of significant heterogeneity between studies without a plausible explanation.
Indirectness of evidence	Is present when there is no available head-to-head comparison between interventions of interest, or when the intervention is assessed for other condition, in a different population, compared with a non-relevant comparator or evaluated for a different outcome than the one of interest.
Imprecision	Presence of large confidence intervals in the analyses.
Publication bias	Assessed through the funnel plot analysis and is likely present when there are few published studies sponsored by the industry.
Factors That Might Increase the Quality of Evidence	
Large magnitude of the effect	Consistent estimates increase the confidence in the obtained results so that the magnitude of the effect is directly proportional to the strength of evidence.
Plausible confounding	If plausible bias would reduce the magnitude of the effect, the confidence in the results increases.
Dose-response gradient	The presence of a dose-response gradient (i.e. higher the dose, better the response) enhances the confidence in the effect estimate, increasing the quality of evidence.

A considerable benefit of GRADE is the clear and transparent process of switching from evidence to recommendations. When clinicians pay the proper attention to the strength of the recommendations, rather than the evidence only, patients would likely benefit from optimal clinical decisions. It is important to highlight that strong recommendations do not necessarily arise from high-quality evidence, since low-quality evidence can generate strong recommendations and vice-versa.

The two grades of recommendation provided by the GRADE system are *strong* and *weak*. A recommendation is considered strong when the intended effect (e.g. reduction in mortality, quality of life improvement) of an intervention overcome the undesirable effect (e.g. adverse effects) (or not) with a high level of confidence in this result.

A weak recommendation is observed in situations in which the level of evidence is low or when evidence indicates similarities between desirable and undesirable effects. Moreover, factors as ambivalence regarding patients' values and preferences or concerning the use of resources (i.e. cost of intervention) may influence the strength of recommendation (G. H. Guyatt, A. D. Oxman, R. Kunz, et al., 2008; G. H. Guyatt, A. D. Oxman, G. E. Vist, et al., 2008).

FUTURE RESEARCH DIRECTIONS

To ensure that future healthcare users can be assured of receiving appropriate care, healthcare professionals must effectively incorporate the necessary knowledge, skills and attitudes required for evidence-based practice into education programs. In addition to developing competence in the fundamental evidence-based practice steps of 'Ask', 'Acquire', 'Appraise', 'Apply' and 'Assess', developing competence in effectively communicating evidence to others, in particular patients and service users, is an area newly emphasized as requiring additional attention by healthcare educators.

Future research to evaluate other learning outcomes such as clinical decision-making and patient outcomes is warranted. Furthermore, when designing future evidence-based practice interventions, educators should consider trends in healthcare education, such as online learning or mobile device learning.

CONCLUSION

A multifaceted approach that encourages the active engagement of students in the learning process is the best method to develop competences of evidence-based practice. The acquired knowledge, skills, and attitudes allow the healthcare professional to translate evidence into practice, which is expected to improve patients' health outcomes.

This chapter provided an overview of the most effective teaching approaches regarding evidence-based practice in addition to supporting material to assist healthcare students and professionals to integrate evidence into clinical decision-making.

REFERENCES

Alt, D. (2015). Assessing the contribution of a constructivist learning environment to academic self-efficacy in higher education. *Learning Environments Research, 18*(1), 47–67. doi:10.100710984-015-9174-5

Andiwatir, A., & Betan, Y. (2019). Letter to the Editor: Evidence-based practice for nursing profession: Barriers and teaching strategies solutions. Int J Nurs Sci, 6(1), 123-124. doi:10.1016/j.ijnss.2018.11.009

Applin, H., Williams, B., Day, R., & Buro, K. (2011). A comparison of competencies between problem-based learning and non-problem-based graduate nurses. *Nurse Education Today, 31*(2), 129–134. doi:10.1016/j.nedt.2010.05.003 PMID:20817332

Aromataris, E., & Munn, Z. (Eds.). (2017). *Joanna Briggs Institute Reviewer's Manual*. The Joanna Briggs Institute. Available from https://reviewersmanual.joannabriggs.org/

Balshem, H., Helfand, M., Schunemann, H. J., Oxman, A. D., Kunz, R., Brozek, J., ... Guyatt, G. H. (2011). GRADE guidelines: 3. Rating the quality of evidence. *Journal of Clinical Epidemiology, 64*(4), 401–406. doi:10.1016/j.jclinepi.2010.07.015 PMID:21208779

Cheung, M. W., & Vijayakumar, R. (2016). A Guide to Conducting a Meta-Analysis. *Neuropsychology Review, 26*(2), 121–128. doi:10.100711065-016-9319-z PMID:27209412

Evans, D. (2003). Hierarchy of evidence: A framework for ranking evidence evaluating healthcare interventions. *Journal of Clinical Nursing, 12*(1), 77–84. doi:10.1046/j.1365-2702.2003.00662.x PMID:12519253

Fernandez, R. S., Tran, D. T., Ramjan, L., Ho, C., & Gill, B. (2014). Comparison of four teaching methods on Evidence-based Practice skills of postgraduate nursing students. *Nurse Education Today, 34*(1), 61–66. doi:10.1016/j.nedt.2012.10.005 PMID:23107585

Flavell, J. H. (1979). Metacognition and Cognitive Monitoring: A New Area of Cognitive—Developmental Inquiry. *The American Psychologist, 34*(10), 906–911. doi:10.1037/0003-066X.34.10.906

Guyatt, G. H., Oxman, A. D., Kunz, R., Falck-Ytter, Y., Vist, G. E., Liberati, A., ... Group, G. W. (2008). Going from evidence to recommendations. *BMJ (Clinical Research Ed.), 336*(7652), 1049–1051. doi:10.1136/bmj.39493.646875.AE PMID:18467413

Guyatt, G. H., Oxman, A. D., Kunz, R., Vist, G. E., Falck-Ytter, Y., & Schünemann, H. J. (2008). GRADE: What is “quality of evidence” and why is it important to clinicians? *BMJ (Clinical Research Ed.)*, *336*(7651), 995–998. doi:10.1136/bmj.39490.551019.BE PMID:18456631

Guyatt, G. H., Oxman, A. D., Vist, G. E., Kunz, R., Falck-Ytter, Y., Alonso-Coello, P., ... Group, G. W. (2008). GRADE: An emerging consensus on rating quality of evidence and strength of recommendations. *BMJ (Clinical Research Ed.)*, *336*(7650), 924–926. doi:10.1136/bmj.39489.470347.AD PMID:18436948

Hatala, R., & Guyatt, G. (2002). Evaluating the teaching of evidence-based medicine. *Journal of the American Medical Association*, *288*(9), 1110–1112. doi:10.1001/jama.288.9.1110 PMID:12204080

Herner, M. (2019). Perfect Top of the Evidence Hierarchy Pyramid, Maybe Not So Perfect: Lessons learned by a novice researcher engaging in a meta-analysis project. *BMJ Evidence-Based Medicine*, *24*(4), 130–132. doi:10.1136/bmjebm-2018-111141 PMID:30842066

Higgins, J. P., Altman, D. G., Gotzsche, P. C., Juni, P., Moher, D., Oxman, A. D., ... Cochrane Statistical Methods, G. (2011). The Cochrane Collaboration’s tool for assessing risk of bias in randomised trials. *BMJ (Clinical Research Ed.)*, *343*(oct18 2), d5928. doi:10.1136/bmj.d5928 PMID:22008217

Higgins, J. P. T., & Green, S. (Eds.). (2011). *Cochrane Handbook for Systematic Reviews of Interventions Version 5.1.0* [updated March 2011]. The Cochrane Collaboration. Available from www.handbook.cochrane.org

Horntvedt, M. T., Nordsteien, A., Fermann, T., & Severinsson, E. (2018). Strategies for teaching evidence-based practice in nursing education: A thematic literature review. *BMC Medical Education*, *18*(1), 172. doi:10.118612909-018-1278-z PMID:30055612

Huedo-Medina, T. B., Sanchez-Meca, J., Marin-Martinez, F., & Botella, J. (2006). Assessing heterogeneity in meta-analysis: Q statistic or I2 index? *Psychological Methods*, *11*(2), 193–206. doi:10.1037/1082-989X.11.2.193 PMID:16784338

Hung, H. Y., Wang, Y. W., Feng, J. Y., Wang, C. J., Lin, E. C., & Chang, Y. J. (2019). Evidence-Based Practice Curriculum Development for Undergraduate Nursing Students: The Preliminary Results of an Action Research Study in Taiwan. *The Journal of Nursing Research*, *27*(4), e30. doi:10.1097/jnr.0000000000000298 PMID:30461524

IntHout, J., Ioannidis, J. P. A., Rovers, M. M., & Goeman, J. J. (2016). Plea for routinely presenting prediction intervals in meta-analysis. *BMJ Open*, *6*(7), e010247. doi:10.1136/bmjopen-2015-010247 PMID:27406637

Khan, K. S., & Coomarasamy, A. (2006). A hierarchy of effective teaching and learning to acquire competence in evidenced-based medicine. *BMC Medical Education*, *6*(1), 59. doi:10.1186/1472-6920-6-59 PMID:17173690

Kuster, M., De Tonnac, A., & Papa, S. (2019). How to write a case-report? *Revue Medicale Suisse*, *15*(664), 1699–1702. PMID:31553533

Kyriakoulis, K., Patelarou, A., Laliotis, A., Wan, A. C., Matalliotakis, M., Tsiou, C., & Patelarou, E. (2016). Educational strategies for teaching evidence-based practice to undergraduate health students: Systematic review. *Journal of Educational Evaluation for Health Professions*, *13*, 34. doi:10.3352/jeehp.2016.13.34 PMID:27649902

Langdon, J., Botnaru, D. T., Wittenberg, M., Riggs, A. J., Mutchler, J., Syno, M., & Caciula, M. C. (2019). Examining the effects of different teaching strategies on metacognition and academic performance. *Advances in Physiology Education*, *43*(3), 414–422. doi:10.1152/advan.00013.2018 PMID:31408387

Larsen, C. M., Terkelsen, A. S., Carlsen, A. F., & Kristensen, H. K. (2019). Methods for teaching evidence-based practice: A scoping review. *BMC Medical Education*, *19*(1), 259. doi:10.118612909-019-1681-0 PMID:31296212

Long, J. D., Gannaway, P., Ford, C., Doumit, R., Zeeni, N., Sukkarieh-Haraty, O., Milane, A., Byers, B., Harrison, L. N., Hatch, D., Brown, J., Proper, S., White, P., & Song, H. (2016). Effectiveness of a Technology-Based Intervention to Teach Evidence-Based Practice: The EBR Tool. *Worldviews on Evidence-Based Nursing*, *13*(1), 59–65. doi:10.1111/wvn.12132 PMID:26773417

Mary, S., Julie, J., & Jennifer, G. (2014). Teaching evidence based practice and research through blended learning to undergraduate midwifery students from a practice based perspective. *Nurse Education in Practice*, *14*(2), 220–224. doi:10.1016/j.nepr.2013.10.001 PMID:24189434

Moher, D., Liberati, A., Tetzlaff, J., Altman, D. G., & Group, P. (2009). Preferred reporting items for systematic reviews and meta-analyses: The PRISMA statement. *BMJ (Clinical Research Ed.)*, *339*(jul21 1), b2535. doi:10.1136/bmj.b2535 PMID:19622551

Murad, M. H., Asi, N., Alsawas, M., & Alahdab, F. (2016). New evidence pyramid. *Evidence-Based Medicine*, *21*(4), 125–127. doi:10.1136/ebmed-2016-110401 PMID:27339128

Patelarou, A. E., Kyriakoulis, K. G., Stamou, A. A., Laliotis, A., Sifaki-Pistolla, D., Matalliotakis, M., Prokopakis, E., & Patelarou, E. (2017). Approaches to teach evidence-based practice among health professionals: An overview of the existing evidence. *Advances in Medical Education and Practice*, *8*, 455–464. doi:10.2147/AMEP.S134475 PMID:28740443

Ramis, M. A., Chang, A., Conway, A., Lim, D., Munday, J., & Nissen, L. (2019). Theory-based strategies for teaching evidence-based practice to undergraduate health students: A systematic review. *BMC Medical Education*, *19*(1), 267. doi:10.118612909-019-1698-4 PMID:31319892

Sackett, D. L., Rosenberg, W. M., Gray, J. A., Haynes, R. B., & Richardson, W. S. (1996). Evidence based medicine: What it is and what it isn't. *BMJ (Clinical Research Ed.)*, *312*(7023), 71–72. doi:10.1136/bmj.312.7023.71 PMID:8555924

Shea, B. J., Reeves, B. C., Wells, G., Thuku, M., Hamel, C., Moran, J., Moher, D., Tugwell, P., Welch, V., Kristjansson, E., & Henry, D. A. (2017). AMSTAR 2: A critical appraisal tool for systematic reviews that include randomised or non-randomised studies of healthcare interventions, or both. *BMJ (Clinical Research Ed.)*, *358*, j4008. doi:10.1136/bmj.j4008 PMID:28935701

Sterne, J. A., Hernan, M. A., Reeves, B. C., Savovic, J., Berkman, N. D., Viswanathan, M., Henry, D., Altman, D. G., Ansari, M. T., Boutron, I., Carpenter, J. R., Chan, A.-W., Churchill, R., Deeks, J. J., Hróbjartsson, A., Kirkham, J., Jüni, P., Loke, Y. K., Pigott, T. D., ... Higgins, J. P. (2016). ROBINS-I: A tool for assessing risk of bias in non-randomised studies of interventions. *BMJ (Clinical Research Ed.)*, *355*, i4919. doi:10.1136/bmj.i4919 PMID:27733354

Tawfik, G. M., Dila, K. A. S., Mohamed, M. Y. F., Tam, D. N. H., Kien, N. D., Ahmed, A. M., & Huy, N. T. (2019). A step by step guide for conducting a systematic review and meta-analysis with simulation data. *Tropical Medicine and Health*, *47*(1), 46. doi:10.118641182-019-0165-6 PMID:31388330

Wells, G., Shea, B., O'Connell, D., Peterson, J., Welch, V., Losos, M., & Tugwell, P. (2000). *The Newcastle–Ottawa Scale (NOS) for Assessing the Quality of Non-Randomized Studies in Meta-Analysis*. Academic Press.

Young, T., Rohwer, A., Volmink, J., & Clarke, M. (2014). What are the effects of teaching evidence-based health care (EBHC)? Overview of systematic reviews. *PLoS One*, *9*(1), e86706. doi:10.1371/journal.pone.0086706 PMID:24489771

KEY TERMS AND DEFINITIONS

Decision-Making: Is the step-by-step cognitive process of making choices by identifying a decision, gathering information, and assessing alternative resolutions.

Evidence: The available body of facts or information indicating whether a belief or proposition is true or valid.

Evidence-Based Practice: The conscientious, explicit, and judicious use of current best evidence in making decisions about the care of individual patients.

GRADE Approach: (i.e. Grading of Recommendations Assessment, Development and Evaluation) is a method of assessing the certainty in evidence and the strength of recommendations in healthcare.

Meta-Analysis: A quantitative, formal, epidemiological study design used to systematically assess the results of previous research to derive conclusions about that body of research.

Problem-Based Learning: A student-centered teaching method in which learners are aroused to develop problem-solving skills while acquiring knowledge in self-directed learning.

PRISMA Statement: The Preferred Reporting Items for Systematic Review and Meta-analysis statement consists of a checklist and a flow diagram and is intended to cover the minimum reporting items of a systematic review and meta-analysis.

PICOS Acronym: (i.e. Population, Intervention, Comparison, Outcome, Study design) Is a mnemonic used in evidence-based practice to frame and answer a clinical or health care related question.

Systematic Review: A type of study design allocated at the top of the hierarchy of evidence pyramid that uses systematic methods to collect data, critically appraise research studies and synthesizes findings.

Teaching Methods: Comprises the different principles and methods used by teachers to enable student learning.

Section 2

Emerging Research and Opportunities

Chapter 5

Bridging Pharmacy Education and Health Humanities:

The Contribution of Narrative Medicine to Pharmacists' Caring Abilities

Afonso Miguel Cavaco
https://orcid.org/0000-0001-8466-0484
Faculty of Pharmacy, University of Lisbon, Portugal

Catarina Martins Pires
Faculty of Pharmacy, University of Lisbon, Portugal

Margarida Pinto Dias
Faculty of Pharmacy, University of Lisbon, Portugal

Cecília Beecher Martins
School of Arts and Humanities, University of Lisbon, Portugal

Teresa Casal
School of Arts and Humanities, University of Lisbon, Portugal

Maria de Jesus Cabral
School of Arts and Humanities, University of Lisbon, Portugal

ABSTRACT

Pharmacy education is largely based on learning elements of disease and the corresponding elements of treatment, using the natural sciences and the biomedical perspective. While this is central for competent pharmacists in working on the research, production, and use of drugs, many professionals deal with people suffering from ill-health. Developing clinical roles requires, besides the traditional pharmaceutical knowledge, the ability to understand illness experiences from the perspectives of patients and significant others. Health humanities provide important resources to link human traits and biomedical knowledge, essential for sensitive and responsive pharmacy practice. The chapter aims to explore emerging opportunities for pharmacists' thinking and working with patients offered by the developing movement of health humanities and narrative medicine.

DOI: 10.4018/978-1-7998-4486-0.ch005

INTRODUCTION

Pharmacists as Professionals Engaged in Caring for Individuals' Health

It is widely accepted that pharmacists have long been recognized as healthcare professionals. From the medieval apothecaries until today, pharmacists have contributed to the well-being of citizens mainly through the preparation and dispensation of drugs and health products to the public.

International organizations, such as the World Health Organization (WHO), state that *community pharmacists are the healthcare professionals most accessible to the public* (World Health Organization, 1997). Being often the first port of call, they are trusted by patients to deal with health matters, pharmacists have developed patient care competencies (Wiedenmayer et al., 2006).

Within the European Union (EU), pharmacists' qualifications are automatically recognized between member states (European Parliament, 2013). The Directive 2013/55/EU Article 45 (#2), amongst other expected competencies, specified the personalized support for patients by those administering their medication, which comprises also the dispensing accountability.

The International Pharmaceutical Federation (FIP) states that pharmacists have to communicate effectively (i.e. clearly, precisely and appropriately) with patients, healthcare staff, supporting staff, carers, family relatives and other clients; also, pharmacists should tailor communications to patients' needs, including demonstrating cultural awareness and sensitivity (International Pharmaceutical Federation, 2012).

These requirements strongly advocate that pharmacists' education should comprise training in the so-called Health and Medical Humanities. These are concerned with healthcare and its engagement with the humanities and arts, incorporating patients and the general public experience (Cole, Carlin, & Carson, 2015).

BACKGROUND

Health and Medical Humanities: An Overview

Over the last few decades, Health and Medical Humanities grew out of Bioethics and brought aesthetic tools to medicine and healthcare education, improving the ability to think and act otherwise about health and illness (Alan Bleakley, 2020).

The acquisition and development of features like empathy towards patients and a deeper understanding and accompaniment of their suffering, regarding each condition, has an important role in caregiving. The need to recognize as well the subjective experience of the healthcare professional, necessary for the promotion of professionals' self-care, including the intersubjective recognition of the patients' position, are essential skills to be developed since undergraduate education (Hojat et al., 2009).

The gradually fragmented 'new medicine' (Antunes, 2012), that came to dominate the medical field, has not promoted a better dialogue with the patient, with his/her experience often being ignored, nor has it given much room for an acknowledgment of professionals' subjective experience of being faced with human suffering and the responsibility to alleviate it.

As Hurwitz and Dakin also suggested, there has been an increasing perception that science by itself is necessary but not enough to completely understand *the interaction between health, illness, and disease* and, therefore, provide quality and patient-centered care (Hurwitz & Dakin, 2009). Medical Humanities (MH) do not reject science but they promote the humanities in order to explore their implications and applications for healthcare.

As Claire Hooker points out, MH were driven by a conscious motivation to bring together *the humanities and creative arts as a necessary supplement to technical medical education, which offered little preparation for the emotion and meaning that are intrinsic to encountering illness, tended to reduce patients to the numbers and body parts of biomedical diagnosis, and subject the sick to the uncaring managerial rationalities of health-care systems* (Hooker, 2014 pp. 213-24).

They represent an area of study that considers the nontechnical aspects of medicine, with three main goals: to study the human aspects of medicine, to connect this with the creative arts and to train better healthcare professionals. In its core, the MH intersects medicine with disciplines from the humanities (Hooker, 2008).

One Approach in Health and Medical Humanities: Narrative Medicine

One of the more significant developments of MH has been Narrative Medicine (NM) (Charon 2006, Charon et al., 2017). NM can be described as a patient-centered approach that has promoted a readjustment of the relational component of the therapeutic praxis to better address human illness, dilemmas, and suffering (Hurwitz, 2015).

It was first defined by Rita Charon as *medicine practiced with the narrative competence to recognize, interpret, and be moved to action by the predicament of others* (Charon, 2001). Narrative Medicine uses reading and writing literary methods to develop narrative competence in healthcare (Charon, 2006), and optimize the use of narratives in diagnosis, therapy, training and decisions outside the standardization in the biological sciences (Charon et al., 2017pp. 69).

Charon proposes the introduction of literary studies in medical training and practice because an appropriate 'listening ear' may not always be developed through conventional healthcare training. The three literary-based skills developed in Narrative Medicine are 'close reading', 'creative/reflective writing', written "in the shadow" of the reading text, and 'close reading' of that creative/reflective writing. Such practices encourage the development of 'attention' and 'representation' skills leading to 'affiliation' (Charon et al., 2017 pp.345-50). The 'listening ear' thus developed will be able to hear all aspects of the patients' communication more effectively, whether transmitted verbally or nonverbally, as clinicians' perceptive attention is enhanced. 'Representation' skills acquired through creative/reflective writing enhance physicians' capacity to better appreciate their patients' dilemmas because *writing, as one form of representation, allows an individual to achieve his or her perception* (Charon et al., 2017 pp. 346). Charon also proposes that the medical field is coming to realize that training carers in narrative skills contribute to the development of more reflective medical practices and better care both for the patient and the carer.

Narrating is one of the means whereby human beings address their perplexities, organize experience, make this shareable with others and memorable over time (Kearney, 2004) It is a dynamic and dialogical process that can be used as a means of communication or of manipulation and control, thus requiring ethical scrutiny (Casal, 2014). Whereas science aims for universal knowledge, narratives are plural, particular and situated in specific circumstances, and their interpretation depends on the teller as well as the listener.

It is precisely their life-likeness and their ability to encapsulate the complexity and uncertainty of particular circumstances that explain why illness narratives are memorable and case studies continue to be used in medical education, for, as argued by Montgomery, *Diagnosis, prognosis, and treatment of illness will go on requiring interpretation, the hallmark of clinical judgment* (Montgomery, 2006; p38). Narratives are also a reminder of how both the telling, with its selection of what to tell and how to tell it, and the interpretation, with its selective attention to details, is infused by individual and collective bias. As noted by Spiegel and Spencer, *Recognition that what one hears in someone else's story can depend on one's own experiences and state of mind can change everything – can be culture change* (Spiegel & Spencer, 2016, p58).

The question, then, is not to seek refuge in a naturalistic perspective that objectifies the patient and overlooks the individual experience of illness but to humbly acknowledge the limitations of science as well as the uncertainty and unpredictably inherent to the intersubjective dimension of the therapeutic relationship (Casal, 2014).

Due to its embodied dimension, and centered in the undeniable body/language reciprocity, the medical encounter is indeed the site of living discourses with open meanings. The interpreting of these discourses requires subtle communication skills since they involve complex prosodic and kinetic cues entailing an alert eye and a listening capacity for attentive interaction (Cabral, Mamzer, Hervé, Beecher Martins, & Charon, 2017).

Health Humanities, Pharmacists and Pharmacy Education

It is well recognized that most of the current pharmacy education is excessively focused on the biological, chemical and pharmacological aspects of disease and treatment, and is overall very technical (Teagarden, 2013; Zimmermann, 2013).

Previous studies found differences in European and USA education concerning patient-centered care (Nunes-Da-Cunha, Arguello, Martinez, & Fernandez-Llimos, 2016). Even so, the clinical focus remains mainly based on pharmacists' understanding of patients mostly as individuals with physical symptoms treated with medication, often forgetting they are human beings with very personal and differentiated experiences and perceptions of their illness and suffering. While biomedical texts cannot teach much about this, literary texts can.

To gain some notion of the use of the humanities in pharmaceutical education and practice, a very brief literature search was carried out using the key terms typically found in health and medical humanities for physician and nursing studies i.e. 'health or medical humanities"', 'narrative medicine'. According to authors such as Angela Woods and colleagues (Whitehead & Woods, 2016), the independent use of the term narrative medicine is debatable as they consider this may be encompassed by medical humanities as such, this expression was also applied.

Using the Boolean operator AND, as well as adding the truncated term "pharm" to the search expression, articles titles and abstracts were searched within the main sciences bibliographic databases (Web of Science, Scopus, and PubMed). Results showed less than one dozen relevant papers (i.e. explicitly including pharmacists and/or pharmacy students), indicating that not much work has been done in this area yet. Still, the papers indicated noteworthy results. It was possible to find two main clusters: one comprising argumentation on the use of narratives and humanities in pharmacy practice or extensive to practice; the other comprised applications and experiences in healthcare education.

As an illustration, studies addressed issues of inappropriate workspace to perform extended pharmacy services (Rapport et al., 2010) and the advantages of using personal narratives to improve pharmacy practice and patient care (Naß, Banerjee, Efferth, & Wohlmann, 2016). It is to be noted that articles show positive educational outcomes, beyond enhanced empathy and compassion, when the humanities were introduced, (Goodman-Snitkoff & Snitkoff, 2006; Teagarden, Assa-Eley, & Nemire, 2013). They also indicate greater effectiveness in responding to illnesses arising from an improved connection between biomedical knowledge and individual meanings of disease on the part of pharmacists (Teagarden, 2013; Zimmermann, 2013).

Of particular relevance were the findings of studies that refer to the impact of medical humanities in healthcare students' interpersonal and interprofessional skills (Ilcewicz, Poirier, & Pailden, 2018; Poirier, Stamper-Carr, & Newman, 2017). The use of literature, cinema, media (podcast) allowed students to interpret and discuss topics in care and ethics, aging and death, personification and stigmatization, amidst other topics.

There was a statistically significant increase in empathy ($p < 0.013$) between paired groups, as well as in the quality of critical thinking and reflective writing associated with greater respect for autonomy, capacity to create relationships, and self-awareness (Ilcewicz et al., 2018; Poirier et al., 2017). Additionally, the positive effects on empathy and academic success of the inclusion of narrative medicine studies were demonstrated through a randomized control trial. The comparison between intervention and control groups of nursing students, who were measured longitudinally (30 months) as to their objective empathic capacity, showed statistically significant differences ($p < 0.05$) immediately, as well as one and a half years after the narrative medicine studies (Yang et al., 2018).

A supplementary search was carried out in periodicals recognized as preferential dissemination outlets for narrative medicine and the medical humanities fields, such as *ARS Medica*, *The Belleview Literary Review*, *The Yale Journal for Humanities in Medicine*. As in the case of the academic papers, the results of non-fictional articles involving pharmacists were low, less than 5%, and have shown both positive and negative accounts. On the positive side, narratives of professionalism, helpfulness, discretion, attention, emotional reading, empathic attitude, positive reinforcement, genuine support, confidence, and soft persuasion, while professionalism embedded within patient acceptance was an overall theme; on the negative side, knowing some drug treatments imply high levels of suffering, narratives of lack of privacy, disregard, disrespect, and distrust were also registered (Case, 2005; Rosenblatt, 2005).

With narrative medicine and illness stories, pharmacists and pharmacy students can begin to perceive disease beyond its physical signs (Teagarden, 2013). Including narrative analysis of texts, movies and other forms of art in pharmacy education can train pharmacists to understand more deeply the plight of their patients and help them develop a broadened view of the illness experiences, making them more empathic and sensible to their patient's conditions and how it affects their daily lives and more aware of their role in the lives of the sick (Zimmermann, 2013).

Narrative medicine and medical humanities can help train better healthcare professionals in general, pharmacists included. Acquiring knowledge in this field and combining it with the technical knowledge pharmacists are equipped with can provide more effective practicing pharmacists, who understand the whole experience of illness and, therefore, are able to provide better advice and counseling (Teagarden, 2013; Vanstone et al., 2016).

NARRATIVE MEDICINE CONTRIBUTIONS TO PHARMACEUTICAL EDUCATION

There are several successful examples of health humanities applications to healthcare professionals' education, more precisely involving narrative medicine approaches.

The pharmacy examples include a study at the University of Wisconsin, Madison School of Pharmacy. Here, a partnership model between first-year students in pharmaceutical sciences and a community of elderly patients was developed. Students' visits were documented in individual writing. Initially, students received training on sensitivity to cope with the elderly, appropriate communication strategies and also practices on medication, blood pressure, and blood glucose measurement. Since students from the first year are not yet equipped with scientific and clinical knowledge, the focus was on an approach more related to care rather than healing.

At the end of the course, students felt that their confidence had increased, including the ability to communicate with the elderly about their health through questions and actively involve them in issues related to their medication. The elderly gave an excellent student assessment regarding students' ability to perform communication, career guidance and health management tasks, especially valuing patient-pharmacist interaction, as well as the genuine interest and young people's concerns about their health, especially in terms of active listening.

Through the reflective questions and experiences, the students had an opportunity to listen to patients' narratives, to put themselves in the place of the elderly and to consider their perspectives, overcoming prejudices they had had before meeting the elderly and so enabling them to build a true partnership. The vast majority also mentioned the importance of listening carefully and with the heart to establish a stable, respectful and trusting relationship with patients as future pharmacists (Martin, Porter, Shawl, & Motl Moroney, 2012).

Another example comes from the elective course entitled "The Heart of Pharmacy", taught at the University of California San Francisco aiming to encourage mutual learning between pharmacy students and faculty members. There were five topics addressed in the course: "Tending to Our Patients", aimed to understand the importance of being dedicated to the patient without any moral judgment; "Tending to Ourselves", involved the recognition of oneself as a conscious and empowering being, having the maximum decision power over ones' own life; a third topic, "Tending to Life Changes", where the objective was to admit and confront the reality of changes that occur throughout life, how those have emotional and physical effects, and how important it is to listen with your heart to be able to overcome situations; the fourth topic, "Tending to Appreciation and Alignment" is proposed to illustrate the intrinsic values of the profession and to remember the powerful and impactful feeling that is giving of oneself to others; finally, the fifth and last "Translating Heart Matters into Practice", aimed at exploring the value of a reflection-based learning in a reliable and stimulating environment and how the concepts can apply in the relationship between the pharmacist and the patient. In summary, students revealed that they grew up both professionally and personally with what they learned in the sessions, recognizing that the daily struggles they experience are not only theirs but also their colleagues' and there is room for mutual support.

Another important aspect mentioned was that this was a unique opportunity to address patients as human beings and not clinical cases, strengthening the idea of the absence of barriers and the need for looking at psychosocial aspects of the relationships with the patient. Finally, the individual awareness resulting from participating in the course was also valued, namely that healing is not just about medication, requiring cognitive and affective skills (Vogt & Finley, 2009).

The Tools of Narrative Medicine

According to the Narrative Medicine approach, healthcare professionals – in this specific case, pharmacists – can become more aware of their patients' experiences of illness if they develop narrative skills. Using Narrative Medicine techniques can be one way to achieve this.

Close Reading and Creative/Reflective Writing Interplay

Medical humanities seek improvement of healthcare providing by humanizing it – this means making it more centered on patients and less on healthcare providers and the technical aspects of the disease. Their goal is to complement the technical knowledge healthcare professionals already have (Duarte, Beecher Martins, & Pereira, 2019; Beacher Martins & Soares, 2019).

Narrative medicine believes that contact with literary texts can help healthcare professionals to better understand their patients' stories. The skills practiced in narrative medicine are close reading, creative/reflective writing written in the shadow of the text, and close reading of creative/reflective writing. Of these skills, this work will focus essentially on close reading, deemed by Rita Charon as the "signature method" of NM (Charon et al., 2017, p157).

The technique of close reading consists of a focused reading that considers the observation of various details and allows attention skills to be developed. This way, healthcare professionals can become more aware of every aspect transmitted by the patient, whether conveyed verbally or non-verbally.

Reflective writing's goal is, briefly, to help healthcare professionals develop the skills they need to represent, in words, that which is observed and felt. And finally, Charon proposes that sharing these written representations with other healthcare professionals and analyzing the texts using not personal references but close reading techniques will help to produce affiliations in those partaking in the healthcare relationship (Beecher Martins & Soares, 2019).

Attention, Representation and Affiliation

When reading a text closely or listening to a patient, the reader must be aware of a series of aspects that will allow him to fully understand what is being said – that includes comprehending what is written or spoken and what is not, and is capable of going beyond words. Paying attention to detail in this manner enhances attention skills (Cabral et al., 2017).

It is clear in narrative medicine that writing about patients in a nontechnical discourse is a good path to perceive them, to understand them more deeply, as well as to understand the caregiver's own emotional response, as healthcare professionals, to the patient's suffering. It is a way to clarify the caregiver's relationship with the patient and, ultimately, to create more empathy and give him more effective medical care. And these two last characteristics are the goal of narrative medicine.

This implies not only using technical knowledge when helping a patient, but combining these with the skills of recognizing and absorbing the experience of the Other (Charon, 2006; Charon, Hermann, & Devlin, 2016)[1].

Attention

Charon proposes 'attention' as the basis of any healthcare giving. From Charon's perspective, before any type of care is given to the patient, the caregiver must listen to the patient's account of events and reflect it back to him.

This requires a kind of attention that is not easy to achieve. Ideally, the "I" disappears, and inner distractions are muted, in a way that the caregiver's concentration is completely turned to the patient. Healthcare professionals must create empathy with their patients in order to understand each patient's psychological state and experience himself what the patient is feeling. And, in the light of the caregiver's knowledge and the empathy created with the patient, the latter gives meaning to what is being told.

Close reading gains importance here as it stimulates the skills required to achieve this kind of attention. With narrative training, we *allow ourselves as readers to be taken up by the author or the text; we donate ourselves – our cognitive machinery, our affective responsiveness, our powers of interpretation, our memories of other texts – to the demands of form and plot* (Charon, 2006).

And when this attention capacity is developed in healthcare professionals, they not only understand their patient's situations more accurately but also help them in the search for personal meaning (Charon, 2006).

Representation

According to Charon, 'representation' – achieved through creative/reflective writing written in the shadow of the text – can be defined as the process of the narrative writing that takes place after this state of attention. Therefore, there is a reciprocal connection between attention and representation.

Memories, sensations, and perceptions are "metabolized" and gain a new form when a creative/reflective writing exercise, written in the shadow of the text that has been analyzed through close reading. Thus, the writing produced is not a product of the writer's imagination exclusively but arises from the experiences lived by its author.

'Representation' is, therefore, a consequence of attention. However, without representation, attention cannot be fully achieved, as *no perception occurs without representation* (Charon, 2006). This representation, especially if written, which allows for thoughts and emotions to be articulated and externalized, enables the writer to discover new aspects of his experience that were not clear before they were written down. By conferring a form to the experience, s/he can examine it from other points of view (Charon, 2006).

Affiliation

Narrative medicine encourages healthcare professionals to represent their patients and themselves in a richer way, through the power of creative or reflective writing, where the "I" stands out more than in any other form of writing (for example, hospital charts or case reports). This kind of writing captures personal thoughts and other more metaphorical dimensions of communication both for patient and healthcare professional.

It goes beyond technical and biological experiences and allows the healthcare professional not only to be in touch with the emotional dimensions of the relationship with his patient but also to notice new aspects of the patient in further meetings. In narrative medicine workshops, the participants read their reflective/creative writing texts aloud to small groups and these texts are analyzed using close reading techniques (Duarte et al., 2019; Beecher Martins & Soares, 2019). The recognition of representation offered by this procedure facilitates the capacity to build affiliations.

Acts of attention and representation culminate in action (Charon, 2006). As a result of the narrative work, healthcare professionals can do more for their patients. It allows them to *affiliate into effective dyads of care with individual patients* (Charon, 2006) and also with other healthcare professionals. Professionals are no longer just observers of the patient's plight – we are part of it. Professionals attend to their patients, represent it and create an affiliation with them. If pharmacists listen closely to our patients, they become newly attuned to ourselves.

Close Reading and Pharmacy Practice

Pharmacists are most times bounded to practice requirements and guidelines. Education itself follows numerous timings, protocols, and rules. These are useful in practice and many times legally necessary, such as when dealing with severe conditions (e.g. Alzheimer's) or when handling drugs (e.g. opioids).

However, besides compliance with best clinical practice, demanding situations provide important opportunities to understand the role of pharmacists when dealing with suffering patients and caregivers. In this chapter we will look at how the management of Alzheimer's disease and opioids use in chronic pain will be addressed using a narrative medicine perspective, respectively through the close reading of the book by Wendy Mitchell *Somebody I Used to Know* and the 2014 drama film *Cake* (directed by Daniel Barnz).

These two examples aim to illustrate what health humanities may add to pharmacists' education and practice. For other examples and approaches, we suggest the papers by Teagarden (Teagarden, 2013) and Zimmermann (Zimmermann, 2013).

Close Reading Applied to a Book

Wendy Mitchell's memoir *Somebody That I Used to Know* was co-authored by journalist Anna Wharton and published in 2018. It describes in the first person the author's memories, her journey from the moment she becomes aware of the first apparently unspecific signs of dementia up to the present. It also features italicized sections in the second person, in which Wendy addresses her younger self, thus allowing both herself and the reader to perceive how her present decisions are informed by her experience.

In the beginning, both healthcare professionals and the author would believe in other diagnoses. Later Alzheimer's disease was confirmed. The book presents the author's views of her daily life, as a patient living with this disease and the whole adaptive process. Wendy was diagnosed at 54 years of age with early-onset dementia and her life, as she knew it, changed. Her adaptation to the changes brought about by this most feared disease is described in rich, extensive and in-depth accounts of physical, emotional, and intellectual changes experienced by the narrator, constitutes a source of knowledge and learning for healthcare professionals.

The book portrays the unfolding struggle to cope with the difficulties presented to these patients, from professional limitations to relearning how to perform basic daily tasks, such as cooking, personal hygiene and taking medication. This book offers important evidence so that pharmacists' may effectively contribute to the wellbeing of Alzheimer's patients.

Somebody That I Used to Know – Book Overview

The memoir illustrates the narrator's long path from the first signs and symptoms to Alzheimer's diagnosis of dementia. This led to contacts with various healthcare professionals. These were not always positive experiences and included instances of not feeling recognized as a human being, through the devaluation of her discourse and her descriptions of physical symptoms and cognitive impairment, which prevented an earlier accurate diagnosis.

Family doctors were informed that forgetfulness remained constant, with a significant worsening over time, including situations where the narrator couldn't remember usual names and places, but this was considered a result of aging, making the narrator believe that her complaints were not being given sufficient attention or credit.

After several appointments with different professionals, resulting in various diagnoses and treatments, she was referred to a clinical psychologist, which gave her a sense of relief because she felt that her case was finally receiving attention: the clinical psychologist was attentive and concerned, being the first to mention the possible diagnosis of early dementia. Nevertheless, she resumed the normal activities of her daily life, though significant symptoms were worsening. She felt as if her brain and the rest of the body were not communicating.

Two years after several consultations with multiple healthcare professionals, a neurologist refers to the definitive diagnosis of dementia. The narrator refers to the pity she felt as she was looked at, which made her uncomfortable and anxious. The narrator shares with the reader the anger of feeling abandoned and discarded by the NHS, where she had worked for over twenty years. In a meeting with an occupational health consultant, it was hard to figure out what her job options would be. The narrator did not suffer from a physical disability and believed minimal adaptions in work conditions would suffice.

However, at the meeting she realized there was no interest in possible workplace adaptations; instead, the suggestion made and even almost forcibly imposed upon her was early retirement for health reasons, which generated a deep upheaval and sadness for not feeling heard or seen as a human being able to work. As a result of feeling abandoned by healthcare professionals, the narrator always tried to be proactive in seeking information about the impact of dementia on one's life, with special attention to new scientific discoveries of possible treatments.

Increasingly bothered by the city noise, after receiving her diagnosis the narrator moved home to a quieter location, where one of the daughters lived. This move proved to be very challenging and difficult because sometimes she felt as if losing the control and independence that she had had and treasured before. She felt she might not recognize her own home from the outside and marked tiles were placed on the front door. Many other strategies (described next) were used in-doors to reduce disorientation and panic.

The pharmacist can be involved as a helpful member of the primary healthcare team, in close and frequent contact with most patients, able to provide counseling regarding memory and provide advice and reminders on issues beyond medication.

Book Deliverables for Pharmacists' Education and Practice

In cases where the patient decides to continue living on his/her own as long as possible, there are several factors to be considered. The patient herself must recognize that it is extremely important to stay healthy and active, both physically and psychologically. Regular exercise in the form of walking is important but keeping the same path.

A well-balanced diet is the foundation of healthy living. To be able to maintain a daily and stable routine the patient can resort to various techniques:

- Annotate on a notebook, whiteboard, or electronic device, e.g. phone or tablet, a list of important information to remember later, such as appointments (with family and friends), phone numbers, ideas, etc.
- Identify with labels and/or photographs the content of house divisions, cabinets, drawers to minimize the anxiety of not knowing what to find or where the objects are stored.
- Make visible and easily accessible the most needed objects such as the mobile phone, wallet, keys, and medication. It may also prove useful for neighbors to have a set of keys.
- In case of leaving home always have your main information with you, such as name, address, emergency contacts and information about the disease you have. In some cases, there are patients who have bracelets or necklaces.

For those who live alone, as happens with Wendy, it makes sense, whenever possible, to have a good support network, whether it is family, friends, neighbors, or healthcare professionals. These are people who can help with everyday tasks and also with whom the patient can talk and stay in touch regularly to combat the feeling of loneliness that dementia can confer.

If the presence of close and known people willing to help is not possible, there is always the alternative of online associations, forums, and communities that can prove to be a solid foundation for support for those who are alone.

Just as important, Alzheimer's patients should stay mentally active. Performing activities such as doing crossword puzzles, reading books and even some creative activities such as painting, sewing, drawing, or playing a musical instrument are important.

Contact with other people can also help if there is not much noise and confusion and for some patients, it is useful and beneficial to participate in groups for dancing. In Wendy Mitchell's case, she refers that making Sudoku all mornings while drinking tea, playing solitaire on her iPad, and Scrabble with her daughter Sarah and the friend Anna are important activities. All invitations accepted to speak or just be a listener at conferences and meetings help her exercise the brain and keep up busy to "beat" dementia.

Being organized is demanding, but it is another way to get over the disease and be able to run your life. At the beginning of each week, the narrator prints daily instructions and activities as well as emails to know where she needs to go and what she needs to do. This organization is very useful when she has to travel: the transportation and route schedules are printed along with photos of the places where she will pass so that when arriving it is easier to recognize the sites. In hotels where she is staying, she keeps the curtain open and a post-it on the table to remember where she is and why, so that when waking up in the morning, or even In the middle of the night, she doesn't feel afraid or in panic.

Other important topics mentioned in the book are oral hygiene, nutrition, and medicines. As a consequence of forgetfulness associated with dementia, the patient likely keeps remembering less and less of oral hygiene. In the bathroom, an explanation can be placed next to the brush and paste on how they should be used and why. An electronic toothbrush can also prove to be more useful as it does not involve as much movement coordination. Also, setting alarms to remember and play a favorite song during brushing may help to focus and know that during that time you should brushing teeth. If possible, caregivers should provide a relaxed environment for mealtimes so that it does not involve pressure. In Wendy's case, the strategy to remember meals is to set alarms, since she is living alone and without a partner who can help her with basic needs.

For pharmacists, an extremely relevant and important part of the daily lives of patients with dementia is taking medication. Besides dementia medication, patients often take drugs for other conditions such as hypertension and diabetes, which, if not taken, can lead to more serious consequences. In case there is no caregiver or someone to follow this daily routine, again alarms on a device may prove useful in reminding the need to take the right medication at the right time.

The pharmacists and/or the caregiver should also regularly monitor parameters like blood pressure, blood glucose, and cholesterol. If the pharmacy is committed to follow and help dementia patients it would be relevant to create and develop a database with flagged users that could send automatic messages to remind medication schedules. Wendy describes in the book how to use various alarms on the iPad as a way of remembering the time when she must take the medicines.

Close Reading Applied to a Film

The Narrative Medicine method can be used when reading a film which helps to explore every dimension of the contact between patient and healthcare professional.

Applying Narrative Medicine to films is possible because, as described by Cecilia Beecher Martins and Marta Soares, *as in literature, the observation of the human condition is an essential attribute of filmmakers*(Beecher Martins & Soares, 2019). As they explain, filmmakers produce settings that "prepare the viewer for the unfolding of the story", because if they did not do so, the speed of dialogues and the unwinding of the story would be too fast and the viewer would feel lost in the narrative.

As recognized film scholar Timothy Corrigan defends, all the elements of *mise-en-scène* are carefully managed to produce a predetermined effect in the audience (Corrigan, 2012). Corrigan, as well as David Bordwell and Kristen Thompson, have developed visual literacy analysis techniques that allow for the close reading of film stills and excerpts like that presented by Charon for the close reading of literary texts. This justifies the use of close reading of films in the narrative medicine context.

Like the examination of a narrative applying close reading, close reading applied to films has the same purpose and effect – to look closely at details, develop attention skills and, ultimately, to transport these skills to clinical practice developing a patient-centered attitude and an inclusive empathy. In fact, work is being done to determine if applying narrative method techniques to film stills and scenes that focus on the caregiver-patient relationship can enhance patient-centered care (Brett-MacLean, Cave, Yiu, Kelner, & Ross, 2010; Duarte et al., 2019; Beecher Martins & Soares, 2019; Zimmermann, 2013).

Cake – Film Overview

The film's main character is Claire Bennett, a former Los Angeles defense attorney. Enduring a life of chronic pain, Claire is reduced to a pill-dependent physically and mentally damaged person: fever and recurrent hallucinations burden Claire's already fragile existence. She becomes fascinated by the suicide of a woman in her chronic pain support group, Nina, who summoned up the courage to put an end to her life. This interest forces her to strike an unlikely relationship with the deceased's widowed husband (Roy), as she uncovers the details of Nina's suicide. While developing a poignant relationship with Nina's husband, she also grapples with her own, very raw personal tragedy.

At the beginning of the film, not much is known about the main character, Claire. She suffers from chronic pain, something known because the movie starts with her in a chronic pain support group, but the causes of this pain are unknown. It seems, temporally, that we start in the middle of her story – we don't know what happened to her and we don't know what will happen from then on. And drawing parallels with the real world and the pharmacist's position every day, this is exactly where she starts her relationship: in the middle of the patient's condition. This movie shows us how there is much more to patient's lives than the maladies they present, and that this should be taken into consideration.

Throughout the film, we must look very carefully at what is conveyed, verbally and non-verbally, to understand how the story began. Attention is needed, just like narrative medicine formulates. Trying to decipher *Cake* encourages the viewer to attain a kind of attention that is similar to what would be beneficial in the pharmacist's daily activity. Claire presents her condition more truthfully in her bodily expression than in her words at the beginning of the film.

Her facial expressions show us, several times, that she is in pain. We see it when she sits, by the way, she stays in a very rigid position when sitting, giving the impression that she is only comfortable that way, the way she moves slowly, these are all signs that she is not comfortable. Close reading is, once again, essential for the understanding of all the non-verbal speech that can be equally or even more important than the verbal one.

Moreover, from the beginning, it is understood that she feels her escape from pain is through the medication she takes. If we apply a superficial/literal reading to Claire in the first part of the film, we will have no sympathy for her, but if we pay close attention, we understand that there is more to her condition than appeared initially.

At the end of the movie, it is easier to understand that superficial glances at patients can offer misleading interpretations and that having close reading skills can enhance attention capacities and much more can be learned about patients' conditions than is revealed at a first glance.

Film Deliverables for Pharmacists' Education and Practice

Films such as *Cake*, with a strong medical component, can be very beneficial for pharmacy students and pharmacists as well. *Cake* is a very good example of how a patient's situation can be very difficult to deal with and how there is much more to the patient's plight than what the pharmacists can see at first glance. There is a slow unfolding of effects that can lead an attentive viewer to question their causes, but the viewer must pay attention to go looking beyond the surface presentation.

At the beginning of the film, it is possible to see that Claire has some medication hidden. A close reading viewer might ask why she has this hidden because to have it hidden must mean she should not have it in the first place. Not taking enough of her medicine means that she has enough to allow her to sleep at night. While the viewer may have some ideas about her medication, it is only later at the Clinic that we get to know Claire is taking opioid medication.

So, we now know what kind of medication she is abusing and, in a pharmacist's head, an alarm rings, because opioids have very specific characteristics and their abuse is rather dangerous. When used continuously they have an addictive nature, causing dependence and tolerance. This means two things: Claire depends on her medicines to relieve her pain but, as she continuously takes them, she starts to develop tolerance.

In order to have the desired effect, she needs a higher dose – so she takes more pills. In doing so, she uses her prescription faster, so she needs more to avoid pain. The problem is not resolved so, when she runs out of pills, she needs to get them anyway – a trip to a pharmacy in Mexico. The pharmacist in Mexico understands the situation, but technical knowledge is not enough to help Claire and the pharmacy scene shows how the pharmacist did not do much more for Claire from the superficial or technical reading of the situation.

Even though the sequence of events that led to Claire's condition is not presented chronologically, in the movie they are revealed when attention is paid to *Cake*'s temporality, a skill developed through close reading. *Cake* has three main subdivisions that connect and reveal, little by little, the real dimension of Claire's problem. We start seeing Claire as a cynical loner who refuses help and prizes superficial relationships over genuine ones. She refuses to engage with people who genuinely care for her. She is in a support group, but she does not want to be there and is extremely offensive. She also has physiotherapy sessions at a pool, but she does not try to get better and is rude to her physiotherapist. She deals with her condition by taking medication and because it gives her instant and easy relief, she doesn't try to make progress in other areas.

This initial presentation of Claire's character and behavior may lead the superficial viewer to overlook the fact that the healthcare professionals looking after Claire do not give her appropriate care – from the support group leader who expelled her without referring her to another professional, to the dispensing nurse whom she could easily bribe to get prescription for her medication and the pharmacist who understood her problems but did not care about them, Claire is lacking real patient-centered care.

Curiously, a turning point, which introduced the second subdivision, happens on the trip to Tijuana; not in the pharmacy but in the restaurant where Claire sees another person (Silvana) as another human being and reaches out to help her. From this point, we see a more vulnerable, honest Claire. She opens a door to her ex-husband (Jason), saying she has been better and requests emotional help by asking him to stay with her until she falls asleep instead of resorting to drugs and alcohol. Claire is not, after all, that emotionless, cold woman we thought at the beginning. She reaches out to Nina's widower, Roy, and wants a real connection, he suffered pain too and they form an understanding as no one else could. The attentive viewer will start to ask, why is she forming a connection with someone who has lost a loved one? Through Roy, we learn she had a son who died, but we only understand how he died when the hit and run driver who crashed into her comes to her house, and she loses all control. After kicking him out of the house she attempts to overdose on opioids. For the first time, we see the true dimensions behind her physical pain.

The third subdivision starts after she tries to overdose on opioids. She makes herself sick but still needs to be hospitalized and is on intravenous drugs which leads her to have constant hallucinations. In these Nina shares her feelings of guilt with Claire about not being able to make a birthday cake for her son. When Claire regains consciousness, she demands that the drip be disconnected. In later scenes, she acknowledges her son's death and starts on the path of recovery. Going off her medication makes this extremely hard for her but now she is motivated and, after facing her past, she really gets on the way to get better.

Looking at these subdivisions and understanding the temporality of the film – there is a past that has led to the present, we see that there were reasons why Claire assumed the path we see her on at the beginning of the movie; that of a self-centered, rich white woman who refused help and kept looking for the easy path until it led her to almost dying. However, the attentive viewer also sees that there were reasons for this and that she did not have attentive healthcare professionals caring for her. In real life, temporality is not easy to analyze but having analyzed it in this context may certainly offer a new skill when looking at real-life cases.

Pharmacists can learn a lot if they close read their patients, if they stand side by side with them in their illness, and not just assume a superior place where they know all about the condition. Moreover, pharmacy students, who do not have contact with patients, can benefit from learning close reading through movies like *Cake*. Through these, they can develop these important skills before they begin their professional life in pharmacy, just like they learn so many technical skills, as Teagarden and Zimmerman suggest. Just like Claire needed better support from the healthcare professionals treating her, pharmacists thus trained can offer more patient-centered care, which can also help them understand that most of the time, behind a rude remark or a suffering face there is someone who needs to be helped – and we must be prepared to help them.

FUTURE PERSPECTIVES

The best way to equip pharmacists with these valuable tools is to include them in their academic training. There is no better place to start developing these valuable skills than the place where all the other more technical skills are developed.

Efforts should be made so that not only pharmacists, but all healthcare professionals have experience of how narrative techniques can assist them – as professionals, as healthcare givers and, ultimately, as human beings, and then reinforce the three core concepts creativity, reflexivity and reciprocity recently identified by Rita Charon for a *narrative transformation of Health and Healthcare* (Charon, 2006).

CONCLUSION

Crossing the humanities with the health sciences can be of enormous benefit for healthcare professionals

0. Using narrative medicine and applying close reading techniques to healthcare professionals' daily lives can greatly improve their caregiving. A patient is not just a person with a disease – he or she is a human being with a condition that needs to be looked at and understood from a more profound point of view.

Cake shows the close reader how a superficial look at someone's life can be misleading and how there is much more in another's story if we look closely at it. Every healthcare professional can benefit from paying close attention to their patients, and pharmacists are no exception. Learning to watch and listen closely to others, to attend to certain details and to represent them, to affiliate them with the perceptions of other healthcare professionals can only be of an incalculable benefit.

Healthcare professionals are technically highly qualified and, if equipped with the tools that narrative medicine offers, can become outstanding caregivers, offering empathy and support that no one else can.

REFERENCES

Antunes, J. L. (2012). A Nova Medicina. (F. F. M. dos Santos, Ed.). Lisboa: Editores, Relógio D'Agua.

Beecher Martins, C., & Soares, M. (2019). Visual Literacy Applied to Film Still Analysis in Medical Training. In Present 40th APEAA (pp. 1–11). Academic Press.

Bleakley. (Ed.). (2020). *Routledge Handbook of the Medical Humanities*. Routledge.

Brett-MacLean, P. J., Cave, M. T., Yiu, V., Kelner, D., & Ross, D. J. (2010). Film as a means to introduce narrative reflective practice in medicine and dentistry: A beginning story presented in three parts. *Reflective Practice*, *11*(4), 499–516. doi: 10.1080/14623943.2010.505713

Cabral, M. D. J., Mamzer, M.-F., Hervé, C., Beecher Martins, C., & Charon, R. (2017). Narrative Medicine: What Discourse adds to Listening. *Anglo Saxonica*, *3*(13), 159–180.

Casal, T. (2014). From Person to Patient: From Patient to Person? In P. Bray & T. Casal (Eds.), *Beyond Diagnosis: Relating the Person to the Patient - The Patient to the Person* (pp. 83–110). Inter-Disciplinary Press.

Case, E. (2005). Getting a Grip. *Ars Medici*, *2*(1), 76–79.

Charon, R. (2001). Narrative Medicine: Form, Function, and Ethics. *Annals of Internal Medicine*, *134*(1), 83–87. doi:10.7326/0003-4819-134-1-200101020-00024 PMID:11187429

Charon, R. (2006). *Narrative Medicine: Honoring the Stories of Illness*. Oxford University Press, Inc., doi:10.7326/0003-4819-146-2-200701160-00021

Charon, R., Dasgupta, S., Hermann, N., Irvine, C., Marcus, E., Colón, E. R., ... Spiegel, M. (2017). *The principles and practice of narrative medicine. The Principles and Practice of Narrative Medicine*. Oxford University Press., doi:10.1080/10410236.2017.1403828

Charon, R., Hermann, N., & Devlin, M. J. (2016). Close Reading and Creative Writing in Clinical Education: Teaching Attention, Representation, and Affiliation. *Academic Medicine*, *91*(3), 345–350. doi:10.1097/ACM.0000000000000827 PMID:26200577

Cole, T. R., Carlin, N. S., & Carson, R. A. (2015). Introducing Medical Humanities. *Medical Humanities: An Introduction*.

Corrigan, T. (2012). *A Short Guide to Writing about Film* (8th ed.). Pearson.

Duarte, M., Beecher Martins, C., & Pereira, P. (2019). *Application of Medical Humanities in Nursing Education - - The Design of Two Studies. 40th APEAA.*

European Parliament. (2013). Directive 2013/55/EU of the European Parliament and of the council of 20 November 2013 amending Directive 2005/36/EC on the recognition of professional qualifications and Regulation. *Official Journal of the European Union*, (354), 132–170. Retrieved from https://eur-lex.europa.eu/LexUriServ/LexUriServ.do?uri=OJ:L:2013:354:0132:0170:en:PDF

Goodman-snitkoff, G., & Snitkoff, L. S. (2006). Use of Enriched Case Studies to Enhance Empathy in Pharmacy Students. *Journal of Pharmacy Teaching*, *13*(2), 5–16. doi:10.1300/J060v13n02_02

Hojat, M., Vergare, M. J., Maxwell, K., Brainard, G., Herrine, S. K., Isenberg, G. A., Veloski, J., & Gonnella, J. S. (2009). The devil is in the third year: A longitudinal study of erosion of empathy in medical school. *Academic Medicine*, *84*(9), 1182–1191. doi:10.1097/ACM.0b013e3181b17e55 PMID:19707055

Hooker, C. (2008). The medical humanities: A brief introduction. *Australian Family Physician*, *37*(5), 369–370. PMID:18464968

Hooker, C. (2014). Ethics and the arts in the medical humanities. In P. Macneill (Ed.), *Ethics and the Arts* (pp. 213–224). Springer., doi:10.1007/978-94-017-8816-8_19

Hurwitz, B. (2015). Medical Humanities: Origins, Orientations and Contributions. *Anglo Saxonica III*, *10*, 10–31.

Hurwitz, B., & Dakin, P. (2009). Welcome developments in UK medical humanities. *Journal of the Royal Society of Medicine*, *102*(3), 84–85. doi:10.1258/jrsm.2009.080383 PMID:19297643

Ilcewicz, H. N., Poirier, T. I., & Pailden, J. (2018). Use of mixed-methods approach to assess the impact of a pre- professional health humanities honors course on developing interpersonal skills. *Currents in Pharmacy Teaching & Learning*, *10*(11), 1456–1465. doi:10.1016/j.cptl.2018.08.010 PMID:30514535

International Pharmaceutical Federation. (2012). *FIP Education Initiatives*. A Global Competency Framework for Services Provided by Pharmacy Workforce. Version 1.

Kearney, R. (2004). *On Stories: Thinking in Action*. Routledge.

Martin, B. A., Porter, A. L., Shawl, L., & Motl Moroney, S. E. (2012). A model for partnering first-year student pharmacists with community-based older adults. *American Journal of Pharmaceutical Education*, *76*(5), 85. Advance online publication. doi:10.5688/ajpe76585 PMID:22761526

Montgomery, K. (2006). *How Doctors Think: Clinical Judgement and the Practice of Medicine*. OUP.

Naß, J., Banerjee, M., Efferth, T., & Wohlmann, A. (2016). Pharmaceutical care as narrative practice? Rethinking patient-centered care through a pharmacist's perspective. *International Journal of Clinical Pharmacy, 38*(6), 1346–1349. doi:10.100711096-016-0391-5 PMID:27766501

Nunes-Da-Cunha, I., Arguello, B., Martinez, F. M., & Fernandez-Llimos, F. (2016). A comparison of patient-centered care in pharmacy curricula in the United States and Europe. *American Journal of Pharmaceutical Education, 80*(5), 83. Advance online publication. doi:10.5688/ajpe80583 PMID:27402986

Poirier, T. I., Stamper-Carr, C., & Newman, K. (2017). A course for developing interprofessional skills in pre-professional honor students using humanities and media. *Currents in Pharmacy Teaching & Learning, 9*(5), 874–880. doi:10.1016/j.cptl.2017.05.004 PMID:29233318

Rapport, F., Doel, M. A., Hutchings, H. A., Wright, S., Wainwright, P., John, D. N., & Jerzembek, G. S. (2010). Eleven themes of patient-centred professionalism in community pharmacy: Innovative approaches to consulting. *International Journal of Pharmacy Practice, 18*(5), 260–268. doi:10.1111/j.2042-7174.2010.00056.x PMID:20840681

Rosenblatt, L. (2005). Case Study Monologue. *Ars Medici, 2*(1), 34–44.

Spiegel, M., & Spencer, D. (2016). Relationality Through Literature. In R. Charon, S. Dasgupta, N. Hermann, C. Irvine, E. Marcus, E. R. Colón, ... M. Spiegel (Eds.), *The Principles and Practice of Narrative Medicine* (pp. 15–36). OUP.

Teagarden, J. R. (2013). Well Connected: Pharmacy Education and the Humanities. *The Journal of Medical Humanities, 34*(4), 477–480. doi:10.100710912-013-9249-1 PMID:23979798

Teagarden, J. R., Assa-Eley, M., & Nemire, R. E. (2013). Illness Performed and Imagined: An elective course using Humanities to teach student pharmacists about illness. *Currents in Pharmacy Teaching & Learning, 5*(2), 120–128. doi:10.1016/j.cptl.2012.09.017

Vanstone, M., Toledo, F., Clarke, F., Boyle, A., Giacomini, M., Swinton, M., ... Cook, D. (2016). Narrative medicine and death in the ICU: word clouds as a visual legacy. *BMJ Supportive & Palliative Care*. doi:10.1136/bmjspcare-2016-001179

Vogt, E. M., & Finley, P. R. (2009). Heart of pharmacy: A course exploring the psychosocial issues of patient care. *American Journal of Pharmaceutical Education*, *73*(8), 149. Advance online publication. doi:10.5688/aj7308149 PMID:20221342

Whitehead, A., & Woods, A. (2016). *The Edinburgh Companion to the Critical Medical Humanities* (S. Atkinson, J. Macnaughton, & J. Richards, Eds.). Edinburgh University Press. Retrieved from http://www.jstor.org/stable/10.3366/j.ctt1bgzddd

Wiedenmayer, K., Summers, R. S., Mackie, C. A., Gous, A. G. S., Everard, M., & Tromp, D. (2006). Developing pharmacy practice - A focus on patient care. *World Health Organization, International Pharmaceutical Federation*, 87. Retrieved from http://scholar.google.com/scholar?hl=en&btnG=Search&q=intitle:Developing+pharmacy+practice+A+focus+on+patient+care#3%0Ahttp://www.who.int/iris/handle/10665/69399

World Health Organization. (1997). *The Role of the Pharmacist in the Health Care System - Preparing the future pharmacist: curricular development*. Retrieved from https://apps.who.int/medicinedocs/pdf/whozip32e/whozip32e.pdf

Yang, N., Xiao, H., Cao, Y., Li, S., Yan, H., & Wang, Y. (2018). Does narrative medicine education improve nursing students' empathic abilities and academic achievement? A randomised controlled trial. *The Journal of International Medical Research*, *46*(8), 3306–3317. doi:10.1177/0300060518781476 PMID:29976109

Zimmermann, M. (2013). Integrating medical humanities into a pharmaceutical care seminar on dementia. *American Journal of Pharmaceutical Education*, *77*(1), 1–8. doi:10.5688/ajpe77116 PMID:23459365

ENDNOTE

1 Details of this method are further described in Charon R, Hermann N, & Devlin M J (2016).

Chapter 6
Building the Pharmacy Workforce of Tomorrow:
Aligning Pharmacists' Education With Society Needs

Ema Paulino
Farmácia Nuno Álvares, Almada, Portugal

Filipa Alves da Costa
Instituto Universitário Egas Moniz, Portugal

Mariana Rosa
Ezfy Lda., Portugal

ABSTRACT

The pharmacist is key in assuring a safe and effective supply of medicines, as well as their responsible use. As a direct provider of services, from primary prevention of disease to therapeutic monitoring, pharmacists work to ensure that the patient's drug therapy is appropriate, the most effective available, the safest possible, and most convenient. This chapter contextualizes the importance of aligning pharmacists' education with societal needs, considering the path to Universal Health Coverage and Sustainable Development Goal 3, and makes the case for investing in the pharmacy workforce of tomorrow. It presents a vision for pharmacy and its place in the healthcare system, linking this vision with a needs-based pharmaceutical workforce transformation program of work.

DOI: 10.4018/978-1-7998-4486-0.ch006

INTRODUCTION

We know that good health is essential to sustain economic and social development, as well as poverty reduction. Therefore, growing attention is being given to promoting access to needed services that maintain and improve health. At the same time, people need to be protected from being pushed into poverty because of the cost of health care (World Health Organization, 2013).

Universal Health Coverage (UHC) means that all people have access to the health services they need, when and where they need them, without financial hardship. It includes the full range of essential health services, from health promotion to prevention, treatment, rehabilitation, and palliative care (World Health Organisation, 2017).

The concept of UHC is firmly based on the 1948 WHO Constitution, which declares health a fundamental human right and commits to ensuring the highest attainable level of health for all (WHO, 1948). This concept, however, has moved higher in the agenda since 2012, when in December 2012, the United Nations General Assembly endorsed a resolution on Global Health and Foreign Policy urging countries to accelerate progress toward UHC as an essential priority for international development (United Nations, 2012).

More recently, in 2015, the 2030 Agenda for Sustainable Development was adopted by all United Nations (UN) member States. It includes 17 Sustainable Development Goals (SDGs), which are the blueprint to achieve a better and more sustainable future for all. They address global challenges such as poverty, inequality, climate change, environmental degradation, peace, and health. All 17 Goals are interconnected, and the UN affirms that in order to leave no one behind, it is important that we achieve them all by 2030. Goal 3 is about ensuring healthy lives and promoting the well-being of all ages and is essential to sustainable development.

To make UHC and Goal 3 of the SDGs a reality, societies need individuals and communities who have access to high-quality health services so that they take care of their own health and the health of their families; policymakers committed to investing in health; but also skilled health workers providing quality, people-centered care.

There is no health without a workforce (Campbell et al., 2013). And we can add that there is no UHC without a competent workforce.

This chapter will start by contextualizing the importance of aligning pharmacists' education with societal needs, considering the path to Universal Health Coverage, and make the case for investing in the pharmacy workforce of tomorrow. We will present a vision for pharmacy and its place in the healthcare system, linking this vision with a needs-based pharmaceutical workforce transformation program of work.

The specific objectives of this chapter are to:

- present a vision for pharmacy and its place in the healthcare system.

- describe how pharmacists contribute to Universal Health Coverage and particularly to SDG 3.
- list the competencies needed for pharmacists to fulfill this vision.
- showcase examples of how pharmacists are making use of these competencies.
- advocate for an international and national needs-based pharmaceutical workforce transformation strategy.

BACKGROUND

Pharmacy and Its Place in the Healthcare System

WHO defines a health system as the combination of all organizations, people and actions whose primary intent is to promote, restore or maintain health. This includes efforts to influence the determinants of health as well as more direct health-improving activities. A health system is, therefore, more than the pyramid of publicly owned facilities that deliver personal health services, and it also includes the social and private sector (World Health Organization, 2007).

Every healthcare system in the world is different, with a wide range of payers and providers models and payment and delivery systems, but one thing is common to all of them: no healthcare system in the world is stable (Smith, 1997).

Although differently across countries, health expenditure has been steadily increasing across the OECD, health spending has typically outpaced economic growth in recent decades. While challenges to health system' sustainability may vary between high, middle and lower-income countries, there are some common issues that every country needs to address in order to achieve citizens' health improvement and health equity, in ways that are responsive, financially fair, and make the best, or most efficient, use of available resources (World Health Organization, 2007).

Although health expenditure has contributed to improvements in health outcomes and has been an important source of economic growth and jobs, the financial sustainability of this upward trend isn't free of concern. Health expenditure is projected to continue to rise in the coming future, mainly due to sociodemographic changes - the aging population and the subsequent increase in chronic diseases and long-term care needs - as well as the impact of new technologies, access to medicines and genetics, and precision medicine (Hurst, 2000; Lorenzoni, Marino, Morgan, & James, 2019; Jones, Valentino, Castro, Fernandes, & Mcguinn, 2018).

Indeed, at a global level, people are living longer and healthier lives. Average life expectancy has increased significantly and sharply over the last decades (Kyu et al., 2018). However, a healthy life expectancy is progressing at a slower pace (Kyu et al., 2018). This fundamental need for good health has inspired the vision that the International Pharmaceutical Federation (FIP) holds and shares with healthcare professionals, with their organizations, and with people worldwide, which is "a world where everyone benefits from access to safe, effective, quality and affordable medicines and pharmaceutical care".

For pharmaceutical scientists, this vision means dedication to discovering, developing, testing, manufacturing, and making available safe and necessary medicines and instruments effective in disease intervention and control.

For pharmacy professionals, it means redirecting their practice to respond to changing needs. Over the past 25 years, pharmacy practice has been moving from being product-focused to being patient-focused (Babar et al., 2018; Hepler & Strand, 1990; Who, 2012).

The pharmacist is key in assuring the safe and effective supply of medicines, as well as their responsible use. As a direct provider of services, from primary prevention of disease to therapeutic monitoring, pharmacists work to ensure that the patient's drug therapy is appropriate, the most effective available, the safest possible and most convenient. Pharmacists are now key players in promoting wellness, preventing disease and contributing to disease management, in close collaboration with other healthcare professionals, so that patients are able to get the best possible results from their health care (International Pharmaceutical Federation, 2019).

Emerging medicines require greater clinical pharmacy input to maximize their safety and effectiveness. And unless the education of clinical pharmacists is fully developed and continually updated, the benefits gained from advances in pharmaceutical research and the development of new medicines will be suboptimal. With all this in mind, we should endeavor to support the development of the pharmacy profession, through practice and emerging scientific innovations, sustained by adequate education and training, in order to meet the world's health care needs and expectations.

PHARMACISTS' CONTRIBUTION TO UNIVERSAL HEALTH COVERAGE AND SUSTAINABLE DEVELOPMENT GOAL 3

In a changing health sector context, the pharmacy profession has a responsibility to identify new opportunities for pharmacy practice, to assess and to test them, and to demonstrate its ability to implement them successfully (Wiedenmayer et al., 2006).

As noted before, it is widely noticed that the role of pharmacist has evolved from that of a compounder and supplier of pharmaceutical products towards that of a provider of services and patient care. And although dispensing of medicines still remains a pharmacy domain, healthcare systems demand from pharmacy a more patient-centered approach in improving access to health care and in closing the gap between the potential benefit of medicines and the actual value realized (Organization, 2011; Wiedenmayer et al., 2006).

Within this context, Figures 1 and 2 depict pharmacy services available at the community and hospital levels, respectively, in countries around the world, based on a survey conducted by FIP in 2017, sent to 103 countries.

Figure 1. Community pharmacy services provided around the globe (data from 74 countries)
Source: International Pharmaceutical Federation, 2017

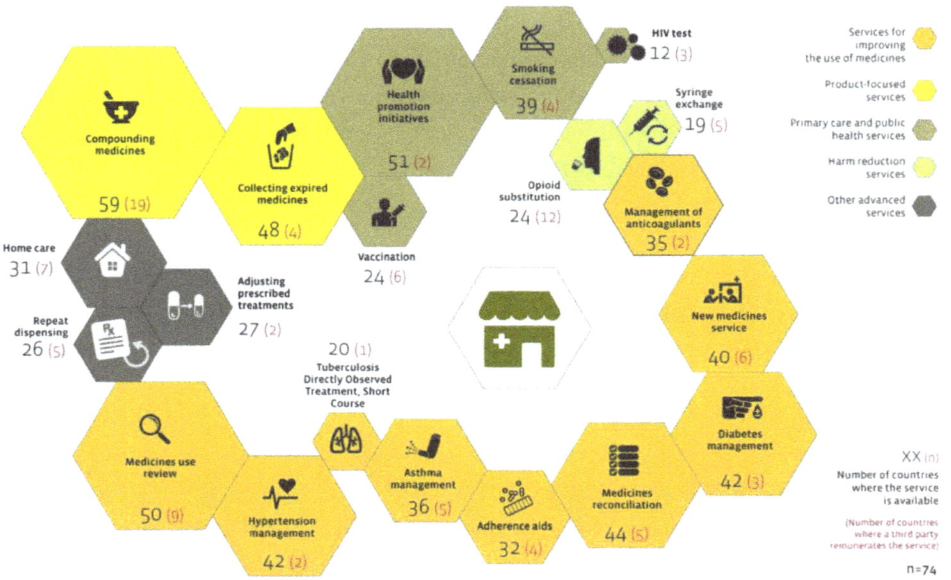

In community pharmacies, several advanced services are common and offered in more than 50% of the surveyed countries and territories, such as medicines use review, disease management programs, as well as the measurement of clinical parameters. Other services like vaccination, needle exchange programs within the context of hard reduction strategies or HIV testing were, at the time of questioning, still available in a smaller number of countries. However, this number has been increasing over the years, as a result of pilot programs and research which has demonstrated their feasibility and added value (Bach & Goad, 2015; Crawford et al., 2016; Kirkdale, Nebout, Megerlin, & Thornley, 2017; Mugo et al., 2017; Papastergiou, Folkins, Li, & Zervas, 2014; Sawangjit, Khan, & Chaiyakunapruk, 2017).

Figure 2. Hospital pharmacy services provided around the globe (data from 72 countries)
Source: International Pharmaceutical Federation, 2017

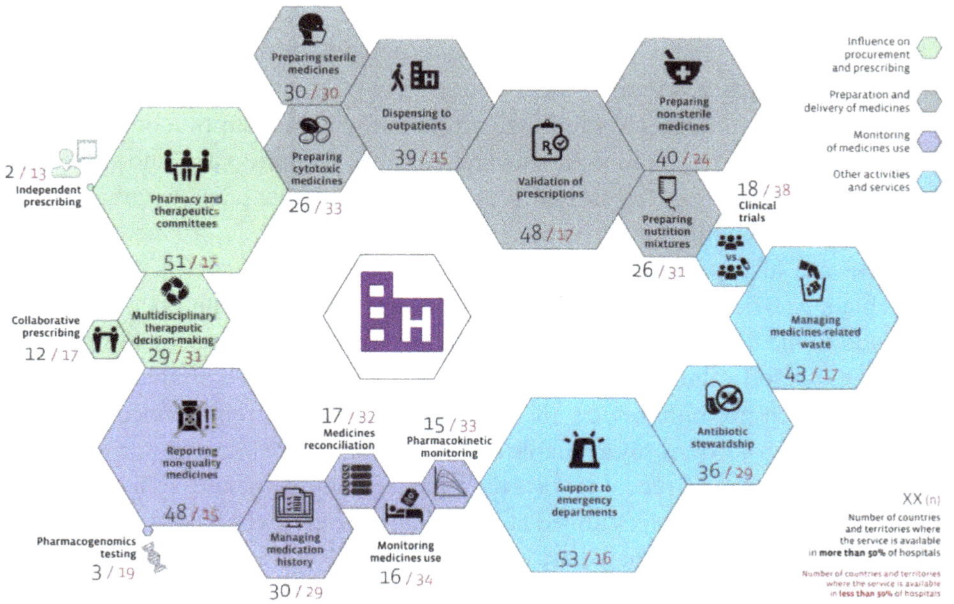

More recent research conducted in this area but restricted to Europe has further indicated the emergence of personalized medicine in community pharmacy (Soares IB, 2020).

Additional research from the same team focusing on medication review practices in Europe has shown the less complex services tend to be more widespread (Imfeld-Isenegger TL, 2019). The first of these papers has however also suggested that although various services exist, the level of implementation of some of these is suboptimal, menacing the contribution of pharmacies to UHC (Soares IB, 2020).

Furthermore, one must highlight that the number of countries where a third party remunerates the services that are depicted in Figure 1 is still quite incipient, which may either mean that they are considered to be covered by the current remuneration system that is in place for community pharmacies (which is mostly dependent on medicines' dispensing volume and/or value), or that they are still not viewed as having a positive return-on-investment by payors. On the other hand, the fact that they are already recognized and paid for in several countries highlights their pertinence and supports the perception that these services are not only needed by patients and societies at large but also able to be provided sustainably and consistently.

In hospitals, the data shows (Figure 2) that the most widely implemented activities are the provision of medicines and support to the emergency department, reporting adverse reactions, and participating in pharmacy and therapeutics committees (International Pharmaceutical Federation, 2017).

Several services aimed at improving the responsible use of medicines are also available in a significant number of countries, as is the case for the application of quality assurance strategies to minimize errors in the administration of medicines, and the implementation of antibiotic stewardship and infection control and prevention strategies. Less implemented are services that refer to direct patient care activities like medicines reconciliation or monitoring medicines use, although there is evidence that these are also gaining momentum due to recognized benefits (Mekonnen, McLachlan, & Brien, 2016; Mueller, Sponsler, Kripalani, & Schnipper, 2012).

To add to the body of evidence of which activities pharmacists are performing, and how these add value to the healthcare system, FIP has been producing a series of reports which not only review the literature for the different services but also gather data which is often only available in "grey literature" or known by professional organizations. The most recent reports have focused on pharmacies as a gateway to care, which describes services aimed at improving self-care; the role of pharmacists in reducing the harm associated with drugs of abuse, including needle-exchange services and methadone programs; the role of pharmacy in promoting medication adherence in the elderly population; services provided by pharmacists which support women in their role of informal caregivers; and the contribution of pharmacists to beating non-communicable diseases in the community (International Pharmaceutical Federation (FIP), 2017a, 2017b, 2018; Sousa Pinto et al., 2019).

Furthermore, an additional report is being prepared on the role of pharmacists in ensuring patient safety, as part of an analysis of the contribution of the profession to the third WHO Global Patient Safety Challenge, related to "Medication Without Harm". This Challenge was formally launched at the Second Global Ministerial Patient Safety Summit in Bonn, Germany on 29 March 2017, and it aims to reduce severe avoidable medication-related harm by 50%, globally, in the next 5 years.

The range of these reports clearly shows the diverse contributions pharmacists can make to achieve Universal Health Coverage and Sustainable Development Goal 3, which in turn should inform curricula development.

It is also of interest to note that pharmacists are starting to practice in less traditional direct patient care settings, as is the case for non-dispensing pharmacists working in primary care and residential, aged-care facilities (Brunisholz et al., 2018; Chen, 2016; Hazen et al., 2018). Specifically, a recent study on the role of pharmacists in primary care units in the UK argued that a definition of the role, with examples of the knowledge, skills, and attributes required, should be made available to pharmacists, primary care teams, and the public, and that training should include clinical skills teaching, set in context through exposure to general practice (Butterworth et al., 2017).

These emerging roles, as well as the new practice settings, present additional challenges for educators. Although we can uphold that many of the required competencies to provide these services will be acquired through post-graduate training, pre-graduate education remains pivotal to ensure that future professionals will be able to permanently seek and assimilate new knowledge and skills.

Competencies Needed by Pharmacists

The concept of competence implies having the capacity to deliver and being able to demonstrate such capacity. It is, therefore, an enhanced application of knowledge, traditionally acquired at the faculty level, and supplemented by practice-based training and experience acquired in real life. These concepts are further detailed in chapters 2 and 7, which we recommend reading. For example, in chapter 2, the FIP clusters are detailed and cluster 5, which refers to experiential education is particularly important in this context (FIP, 2017).

In this section, we will focus on the competencies needed to support the delivery of services required by current societies. In our view and supported by the rationale introduced in the previous section of this chapter, there is a common trend in all these services, which is the capacity to contribute to medication optimization and achieve improved patient outcomes. This implies having a strong focus on clinical pharmacy and pharmacotherapy, also in some contexts referred to as pharmaceutical care. These core areas are common to direct patient care, regardless of the setting, hence applicable to all levels of care provision, including primary care, hospital care and highly specialized care. There are various competencies needed across the full spectra of the activity of these pharmacists, which must be aligned with the patient pathway and the policy priorities established. This means that not only we should invest in treatment but also prevention.

To achieve the needed competencies to enhance medication safety, pharmacists need to practice in an environment with a safety culture (Cordina, 2019). However, it has been shown that safety may not be promoted in isolation, so to achieve safe medication use, the educational transformation must be conducted across various healthcare degrees, both at the undergraduate level and throughout the continuous professional development period. Focusing on the pharmaceutical workforce, to achieve safe medication use, one of the competencies must be around clinical pharmacy but another one is surely interprofessional collaboration. Contrasting with the clusters described in chapter 2, this competence is deeply related to cluster 2 - professional skills mix.

A recent editorial has captured a patient experience in an environment where information recording and sharing practices were suboptimal, clearly showing the impact on the patient level (van Mil, 2019). This implies an additional required competence focusing on information use, documentation and sharing; which is also related to cluster 7 referred to in chapter 2 – quality assurance, although applied to practice and not necessarily to education. For greater detail on drug information, we refer to chapter 3.

Various classifications may be proposed to group the core competences needed by the pharmaceutical workforce to provide services aligned with societal needs (Table 1), which we have identified as being centered around the clinical pharmacy. We propose one possible classification, adapted from elsewhere, but defend that it is not the grouping per se that is central, but the content (American College of Clinical Pharmacy, 2008) (Girvin B, 2018).

Table 1. Core competencies for pharmacists to meet societal needs

Scientific skills	•Strong knowledge about the disease and medicines' mechanism of action. •Solid knowledge about medical terminology. •Strong knowledge of pharmacological interactions and adverse drug reactions (ADRs).
Personal skills	•Communication with patients, medical staff and communities in general. •Decision-making. •Critical thinking. •Problem-solving. •Teamwork.
Professional skills	•An adequate response to medical emergencies, including first aid. •Therapeutic planning and therapeutic drug monitoring. Evaluation and interpretation of laboratory and physical data. •Patient assessment and counseling. •Pharmacokinetic monitoring. •ADR monitoring. •Medicines management and medication review. •Identification and management of medication safety. •Provision of education and information about medicines.

We also defend that the manner through which the professional organizations leading the profession to ensure these competencies are in place will have a major impact.

When talking about competences, it is important to refer to the competence domain, but also the various elements included in such a domain. This exercise is particularly useful for planning career paths, thinking about the individual pharmacist, and for planning competency assessments, thinking from the regulator's perspective.

Table 2. Competency domains and elements of these competencies

Competency Domain	Elements of the Competency
I - Direct patient care	• Assess patients, including identifying and prioritizing patient problems and medication-related needs. • Evaluate drug therapy for appropriateness, effectiveness, safety, adherence, and affordability. • Develop/initiate therapeutic plans and address medication-related problems. • Follow up on and monitor the outcomes of therapeutic plans. • Collaborate with other members of the health care team to achieve optimal patient outcomes across the continuum of care. • Apply knowledge of the roles and responsibilities of other health care team members to patient care.
II - Pharmacotherapy Knowledge	• Demonstrate and apply in-depth knowledge of pharmacology, pharmacotherapy, pathophysiology, and clinical signs, symptoms, and natural history of diseases and/or disorders. • Locate, evaluate, interpret, and assimilate scientific/clinical evidence and other relevant information from the biomedical, clinical, epidemiological, and social-behavioral literature. • Use scientific/clinical evidence as to the basis for therapeutic decision-making. • Possess the knowledge and experience commensurate with certification in one or more Board of Pharmacy Specialties. • Maintain and enhance pharmacotherapy knowledge, including recertification or other appropriate methods of self-assessment and learning.
III - Systems-based care and population health	• Use health care delivery systems and health informatics to optimize the care of individual patients and patient populations. • Participate in identifying systems-based errors and implementing solutions. • Resolve medication-related problems to improve patient/population health and quality metrics. • Apply knowledge of Pharmacoeconomics and risk-benefit analysis to patient-specific and/or population-based care. • Participate in developing processes to improve transitions of care. • Design quality improvement processes to improve medication use.
IV - Communication	• Communicate effectively with a) Patients, caregivers, families, and laypersons of diverse backgrounds; b) Other health professionals and stakeholders. • Provide clear and concise consultations to other health professionals. • Develop professional written communications that are appropriate to the audience. • Use verbal communications tailored to varied clinical and patient-specific environments. • Communicate with appropriate levels of assertiveness, confidence, empathy, and respect.
V- Professionalism	• Uphold the highest standards of integrity and honesty. • Commit to a fiducial relationship with patients, always working in their best interests. • Serve as a credible role model/leader for students, trainees, and colleagues by exhibiting the values and behaviors of a professional. • Advance clinical pharmacy through professional stewardship, training
VI - Continuous professional development	• Commit to excellence and lifelong learning. • Demonstrate skills of self-awareness, self-assessment, and self-development. • Identify and implement strategies for personal improvement through continuing professional development. • Provide professional education to students, trainees, or other health professionals. • Maintain Board of Pharmacy Specialties certification to ensure that therapeutic knowledge is up to date.

This has been the approach taken by the American College of Clinical Pharmacy, introducing six competency domains. Given the relevance of these domains and alignment with what we are defending, we present in greater detail these six domains and the elements contained in each of those (Table 2) (Saseen, 2017).

As may be seen, some of the issues previously addressed are encompassed in this table, namely the focus also on prevention (see domain III) and on treatment (see domains I and II). The strong focus on medication safety is visible in domains I, II and III, but also aspects referring to interprofessional communication and the use of information systems in place are acknowledged in domain IV. Finally, considering we are dealing with an ethically regulated profession where individuals and communities need to be respected and their rights preserved, other competency areas arise as a foundation for all care provided (domain V).

The constant evolution of science and the growing emergence of innovative therapies makes domain VI more and more important as constant updating of knowledge is a prerequisite to excellence in the delivery of clinical pharmacy services.

In Portugal, a competency framework for pharmacists working in different settings was developed by the Pharmaceutical Society in 2016. It is a professional development model that includes the certification of competences, through the organization of development pathways based on the concept of pharmaceutical competences. The intention is to use this competency model as a tool for identification, assessment, and certification, in line with the evolution of the profession.

Specific, dedicated competency frameworks were developed for community pharmacy, hospital pharmacy, pharmaceutical industry, and regulatory affairs. The model proposes that pharmaceutical competencies can then be grouped and lead to the application for a specialization title in each professional area, without prejudice to additional requirements from the respective colleges.

Given that the processes to confer the specialist titles, except for community pharmacy, were already in place before the development of these competency frameworks, there is now a need to align both charters. Whilst the specialization title recognizes the level of expertise of a pharmacist working in a certain practice setting, competences can be more transversal, in that they can be present and necessary in a transversal manner, as is the case for clinical pharmacy in the context of direct patient care.

Showcasing Pharmacy Services

We often contend that practice evolution and changing healthcare-system requirements have to inform pharmacy curricula development and revision (Nunes-Da-Cunha, Arguello, Martinez, & Fernandez-Llimos, 2016). However, we can also state that emerging pharmacy services, although driven by patient needs, are inspired by current competences provided by Faculties of Pharmacy.

In Portugal, pharmaceutical care provision in community pharmacies was first legislated in 2007. A total of eight services that could be provided by pharmacies was listed: homecare assistance, administration of first aid assistance, administration of medicines (e.g. via intramuscular or subcutaneous routes), the utilization of auxiliary means of therapeutic and diagnostic (including those provided by other healthcare professionals), administration of vaccines not included in the National Vaccination Plan, pharmaceutical care programs, engagement in health information campaigns, and collaboration in health education programs.

This legislation was further updated in 2018, expanding on the number of services that can be provided by pharmacists, namely: medication adherence interventions, medication reconciliation, multicompartment aids service, educational interventions for medical devices, and point of care testing for HIV, HBV and HCV.Some of these new services implied pharmacists' accreditation by the Pharmaceutical Society, as was the case for the administration of medicines and vaccines.

In hospital pharmacy, the recent publication of the Pharmaceutical Career diploma (Decree-Law nº 108 and 109/2017, August 30th) represents an important milestone for the profession, since it underlines the high degree of training (pre and postgraduate) and specialization required to perform the respective roles. These include medicines and other health technologies selection, acquisition, storage, and distribution, the implementation and monitoring of the drug policy as defined by the Pharmacy and Therapeutics Commission, and emerging, patient-centered services such as discharge consultations.

We chose to showcase one pharmacy service in the community setting and another in the hospital setting, which illustrates the breadth of pharmacists' activities.

Point-of-Care Testing

Point-of-care testing is a regular service provided by all pharmacies throughout the country. The range of services available varies, but glycemia, weight, blood pressure and total cholesterol are almost universal. Other services are progressively being implemented, namely full lipid profile, HbA1c, INR, etc.

Although point-of-care testing may be provided as a stand-alone service, it is increasingly being recognized to monitor medication effectiveness and safety, as well as to detect some specific diseases early on. To this end, it usually has to be part of a wider evaluation that also considers other indicators and risk factors, including medical history (Sousa Pinto et al., 2019).

Competences needed for this service include many of those referred to above in Table 2, particularly in Domain I, II and IV, apart from Domains V and VI, which are transversal.

Medication Reconciliation Within a Home Hospitalization Unit

Home Hospitalization projects aim to promote patient discharge from hospitals and to prevent re-admissions. In a pioneer project in a hospital in Almada, pharmacists were included in the Home Hospitalization Unit to perform medication reconciliation.

The pharmacists' intervention also included assistance in the storage of medication, identification, and collection of expired drugs, and interventions to enhance adherence to prescribed treatment (Brito, Simões, Costa, & Alcobia, 2016).

Although innovative in Portugal, there is international evidence that supports the expansion of this role, particularly as it reduces unnecessary health care utilization and cost, but more importantly benefits the patient, who remains healthy at home following a hospitalization (Novak, Hastanan, Moradi, & Terry, 2012).

Again, in this case, we can see how competences from Domain I, II and IV mentioned in Table II are relevant and applicable.

As with these examples, and as we identify further pharmacy services like the ones included in Figures 1 and 2, we can most often conclude that all Competence Domains as depicted in Table 2 are required when developing such services.

A NEEDS-BASED PHARMACEUTICAL WORKFORCE TRANSFORMATIONS STRATEGY

Independently of the competency framework that is considered, investing in the development of an adaptable, flexible, and competent pharmaceutical workforce contributes towards achieving UHC and the SDGs, as well as strengthening health systems.

Transforming the pharmaceutical workforce around the world requires a global vision with clear and consensus-based objectives consistent with global health strategies. This vision needs to be translated into concerted actions and engagement at the country-level in order to impact significantly on better population pharmaceutical healthcare, as suggested by the FIP Workforce Transformation Program.

In 2016, the International Pharmaceutical Federation adopted a transformative workforce roadmap, which sets out milestones and outcomes for education and workforce development of pharmacists and pharmaceutical scientists, driven in cooperation with our members and partners, and linked directly and clearly with a global vision for transforming pharmacy.

FIP now urges each country to develop its needs-based, national workforce development strategies, workforce planning, and actions, recommending that they develop this national roadmap in four phases:

Phase I – Create a workforce Vision: Development must be based on needs and every country has its own distinct needs and health system circumstances, so firstly, comprehensive identification of the country-specific workforce development needs must be conducted, through a comprehensive needs assessment and situational analysis process. In addition to a National Workforce Needs Report, the key outcome from this stage is a National Workforce Development Vision.

Phase II – Commit to the Vision: Committing to the Vision created in Phase I requires the full support, engagement, and advocacy of all national pharmacy and health stakeholders. Therefore, in this phase, the promoter should garner advocacy and evidence-led engagement through mechanisms as discussion and briefing papers, designing high-level national leadership events, and access to expertise.

Phase III - Carry out the Vision: One of the most important outcomes is to convert the vision into a sustainable and practical action plan. This action plan should be used to prioritize and achieve the vision in a stepwise fashion, identifying solutions and mechanisms for development and implementation to address selected priorities.

Phase IV – Deliver the Vision: By Phase IV, implementing solutions for the national workforce development priorities should be underway. During this phase, the vision and action plan should be revisited to re-identify new priorities and renew the commitment to transforming the national workforce.

As the authors see it, in Portugal, this is an endeavor for the Pharmaceutical Society to take on, considering its self-regulatory role within the context of a public health defense mandate. However, this cannot be done in isolation, and we suggest that the Education and Practice Platform (Chapter 7) has a role to play in this program of work, given its intersectoral representation.

Additionally, considering that the contribution of pharmacists is part of a larger puzzle which involves other members of the healthcare team to achieve UHC, we suggest that interprofessional initiatives should take place to better coordinate and integrate care, whilst ensuring that patients are empowered to take on a greater role in their process of care.

CONCLUSION

There is no health without a workforce. And there is no Universal Health Coverage without a competent, fit for purpose workforce. Pharmacists are important members of the healthcare team, as they bring specific expertise to the table related to the best use of health technologies, namely medicines. In addition to this traditional role, pharmacists have been taking up new responsibilities, driven by people's needs, and inspired by current competences.

The alignment of pharmacists' education with societal needs, considering the path to Universal Health Coverage, is imperative for the profession, if we are to remain relevant within a changing context. Investing in the pharmacy workforce of tomorrow requires the implementation of a needs-based pharmaceutical workforce transformation program of work, which should be led by the profession itself.

REFERENCES

American College of Clinical Pharmacy. (2008). The definition of clinical pharmacy. *Pharmacotherapy*, 816–817. PMID:18503408

Babar, Z. U. D., Kousar, R., Murtaza, G., Azhar, S., Khan, S. A., & Curley, L. (2018). Randomized controlled trials covering pharmaceutical care and medicines management: A systematic review of literature. *Research in Social & Administrative Pharmacy*. Advance online publication. doi:10.1016/j.sapharm.2017.06.008 PMID:28651923

Bach, A., & Goad, J. (2015). The role of community pharmacy-based vaccination in the USA: Current practice and future directions. *Integrated Pharmacy Research & Practice*. Advance online publication. doi:10.2147/iprp.s63822 PMID:29354521

Brito, A., Simões, A., Costa, F. A., & Alcobia, A. (2016). Revisão e reconciliação terapêutica em hospitalização domiciliária. *IX Congresso Nacional da APFH (Associação Portuguesa de Farmácia Hospitalar): Segurança & Inovação–Pilares do Futuro*.

Brunisholz, K. D., Olson, J., Anderson, J. W., Hays, E., Tilbury, P. M., Winter, B., ... Parkin, G. (2018). "Pharming out" support: A promising approach to integrating clinical pharmacists into established primary care medical home practices. *The Journal of International Medical Research*. Advance online publication. doi:10.1177/0300060517710885 PMID:28789606

Butterworth, J., Sansom, A., Sims, L., Healey, M., Kingsland, E., & Campbell, J. (2017). Pharmacists' perceptions of their emerging general practice roles in UK primary care: A qualitative interview study. *The British Journal of General Practice*. Advance online publication. doi:10.3399/bjgp17X691733 PMID:28673959

Campbell, J., Dussault, G., Buchan, J., Pozo-Martin, F., Guerra Arias, M., Leone, C., . . . Cometto, G. A. (2013). *A universal truth: No health without a workforce.* Forum Report Third Global Forum on Human Resources for Health Global Health Workforce Alliance and World Health Organization.

Chen, T. F. (2016). Pharmacist-Led Home Medicines Review and Residential Medication Management Review: The Australian Model. *Drugs & Aging*. Advance online publication. doi:10.100740266-016-0357-2 PMID:26961696

Cordina, M. (2019). Preparing the health workforce to enhance medication safety. *Research in Social & Administrative Pharmacy*, 813–814. PMID:30885570

Crawford, N. D., Dean, T., Rivera, A. V., Guffey, T., Amesty, S., Rudolph, A., ... Fuller, C. M. (2016). Pharmacy intervention to improve HIV testing uptake using a comprehensive health screening approach. *Public Health Reports*. Advance online publication. doi:10.1177/00333549161310S116 PMID:26862239

FIP. (2017). *Nanjing Statements.* Obtido em 06 de 12 de 2019, de https://www.fip.org/files/content/priorityareas/

Girvin, B. W. D. (2018). Clinical skills training for pharmacists in general practice. *The Prescriber*, 19–25.

Hazen, A. C. M., de Bont, A. A., Boelman, L., Zwart, D. L. M., de Gier, J. J., de Wit, N. J., & Bouvy, M. L. (2018). The degree of integration of non-dispensing pharmacists in primary care practice and the impact on health outcomes: A systematic review. *Research in Social & Administrative Pharmacy*. Advance online publication. doi:10.1016/j.sapharm.2017.04.014 PMID:28506574

Hepler, C. D., & Strand, L. M. (1990). Opportunities and responsibilities in pharmaceutical care. *American Journal of Hospital Pharmacy*. Advance online publication. doi:10.1093/ajhp/47.3.533 PMID:2316538

Hurst, J. (2000). Challenges for health in member countries of the organisation for economic co-operation and development. *Bulletin of the World Health Organization*. doi:10.1590/S0042-96862000000600007

Imfeld-Isenegger, T. L. S. I. (2019). Pharmacist-led medication review procedures: a survey across Europe. Research in Social and Administrative Pharmacy. doi:10.1016/j.sapharm.2019.11.002

International Pharmaceutical Federation. (2017). *Pharmacy at a Glance 2015-2017*. Author.

International Pharmaceutical Federation. (2019). *Beating non-communicable diseases in the community: The contribution of pharmacists*. Author.

International Pharmaceutical Federation (FIP). (2017a). *Pharmacy as a Gateway to care: helping people towards better health*. Author.

International Pharmaceutical Federation (FIP). (2017b). *Reducing harm associated with drugs of abuse: the role of pharmacists*. Author.

International Pharmaceutical Federation (FIP). (2018). *Pharmacists supporting women and the responsible use of medicines*. Author.

Kirkdale, C. L., Nebout, G., Megerlin, F., & Thornley, T. (2017). Benefits of pharmacist-led flu vaccination services in community pharmacy. *Annales Pharmaceutiques Francaises*. Advance online publication. doi:10.1016/j.pharma.2016.08.005 PMID:27717412

Kyu, H. H., Abate, D., Abate, K. H., Abay, S. M., Abbafati, C., Abbasi, N., ... Murray, C. J. L. (2018). Global, regional, and national disability-adjusted life-years (DALYs) for 359 diseases and injuries and healthy life expectancy (HALE) for 195 countries and territories, 1990-2017: A systematic analysis for the Global Burden of Disease Study 2017. *Lancet*. Advance online publication. doi:10.1016/S0140-6736(18)32335-3 PMID:30415748

Lorenzoni, L., Marino, A., Morgan, D., & James, C. (2019). *Health Spending Projections to 2030*. Academic Press.

Mekonnen, A. B., McLachlan, A. J., & Brien, J. A. E. (2016). Effectiveness of pharmacist-led medication reconciliation programmes on clinical outcomes at hospital transitions: A systematic review and meta-analysis. *BMJ Open*. Advance online publication. doi:10.1136/bmjopen-2015-010003 PMID:26908524

Mueller, S. K., Sponsler, K. C., Kripalani, S., & Schnipper, J. L. (2012). Hospital-based medication reconciliation practices: A systematic review. *Archives of Internal Medicine*. Advance online publication. doi:10.1001/archinternmed.2012.2246 PMID:22733210

Mugo, P. M., Micheni, M., Shangala, J., Hussein, M. H., Graham, S. M., Rinke De Wit, T. F., & Sanders, E. J. (2017). Uptake and acceptability of oral HIV self-testing among community pharmacy clients in Kenya: A feasibility study. *PLoS One*. Advance online publication. doi:10.1371/journal.pone.0170868 PMID:28125699

Novak, C. J., Hastanan, S., Moradi, M., & Terry, D. F. (2012). Reducing unnecessary hospital readmissions: The pharmacist's role in care transitions. *The Consultant Pharmacist*. Advance online publication. doi:10.4140/TCP.n.2012.174 PMID:22421517

Nunes-Da-Cunha, I., Arguello, B., Martinez, F. M., & Fernandez-Llimos, F. (2016). A comparison of patient-centered care in pharmacy curricula in the United States and Europe. *American Journal of Pharmaceutical Education*. Advance online publication. doi:10.5688/ajpe80583 PMID:27402986

Organization, W. H. (2011). *Joint FIP/WHO Guidelines on Good Pharmacy Practice: Standards for quality of pharmacy services. Geneva 2011*. Report.

Papastergiou, J., Folkins, C., Li, W., & Zervas, J. (2014). Community pharmacist–administered influenza immunization improves patient access to vaccination. *Canadian Pharmacists Journal*. Advance online publication. doi:10.1177/1715163514552557 PMID:25364353

Saseen, J. J. (2017). ACCP clinical pharmacist competencies. *Pharmacotherapy: The Journal of Human Pharmacology and Drug Therapy*, 630-636.

Sawangjit, R., Khan, T. M., & Chaiyakunapruk, N. (2017). Effectiveness of pharmacy-based needle/syringe exchange programme for people who inject drugs: A systematic review and meta-analysis. *Addiction (Abingdon, England)*. Advance online publication. doi:10.1111/add.13593 PMID:27566970

Smith, R. (1997). *The future of healthcare systems: Information technology and consumerism will transform health care worldwide*. British Medical Journal Publishing Group.

Soares, I. B. I.-I. T. (2020). A survey to assess the availability, implementation rate and remuneration of Pharmacist-led cognitive services in Europe. Research in Social and Administrative Pharmacy, 41-47.

Sousa Pinto, G., Bader, L., Billberg, K., Criddle, D., Duggan, C., El Bizri, L., ... Laven, A. (2019). Beating non-communicable diseases in primary health care: The contribution of pharmacists and guidance from FIP to support WHO goals. *Research in Social & Administrative Pharmacy*. Advance online publication. doi:10.1016/j.sapharm.2019.10.008 PMID:31668903

United Nations. (2012). *Resolution adopted by the General Assembly on 12 December 2012*. Resolutions and Decisions.

van Mil, J. (2019). Seamless care, do it well or not at all. *International Journal of Clinical Pharmacy*, 1391–1393. PMID:31748966

WHO. (1948). *Constitution of WHO*. Official Records of WHO.

WHO. (2012). The Pursuit of Responsible Use of Medicines: Sharing and Learning from Country Experiences. *The Veterinary Record, 169*(9), 78. doi:10.1136/vr.d5420

Wiedenmayer, K., Summers, R. S., Mackie, C. A., Gous, A. G. S., Everard, M., Tromp, D., & Organization, W. H. (2006). *Developing pharmacy practice: a focus on patient care: handbook*. World Health Organization.

World Health Organisation. (2017). *WHO | What is universal coverage?* Health Financing for Universal Coverage.

World Health Organization. (2007). Everybody business: strengthening health systems to improve health outcomes: WHO's framework for action. *Production*.

World Health Organization. (2013). *Arguing for Universal Health Coverage*. World Health Organization. doi:10.1016/j.memsci.2011.12.046

Chapter 7
Implementation and Evaluation of Team-Based Learning in a Pharmacy Law and Ethics Module

Mara Pereira Guerreiro
CiiEM, Instituto Universitário Egas Moniz, Portugal

ABSTRACT

Team-based learning (TBL) is an active learning strategy based on sequential stages: individual advanced preparation, readiness assurance process, and team application. When adopting this instructional strategy, planning entails consideration about organizing contents, securing the right infrastructure, forming groups, and grading students' work. The first class should be used to cover key aspects, such as explaining how TBL works and why it is being used. Facilitating TBL classes demands communication and organizational skills, in addition to content-expertise. TBL was implemented in a pharmacy law and ethics module. The perspectives of students collected through surveys were overall favorable. These perspectives, together with other favorable indicators, led to TBL maintenance until the current days.

INTRODUCTION

The profile of the 21st-century health care professionals - technically competent, able to independently search and appraising available information, capable of critical and reflective thinking, and able to work collaboratively in teams – is one of the driving forces for changes in the education system. There has been a shift from traditional

DOI: 10.4018/978-1-7998-4486-0.ch007

didactic lectures to instructional strategies that actively involve learners, as well as towards a more interactive and meaningful learning environment.

The main objective of this chapter is to describe the implementation and evaluation of team-based learning (TBL), using the case of a pharmacy law and ethics module.

Educators may find the chapter valuable, as it details the practicalities of using this instructional strategy and discusses implementation issues.

The chapter is comprised of several sections. The background section firstly provides an overview of TBL development. Next, the instructional strategy is described, followed by key issues in planning and implementing TBL, based on the literature. This section finishes with an overview of the impact of TBL.

The second section is about the implementation of TBL in a pharmacy law and ethics module. It offers contextual information about the module, explains TBL operationalization and debate choices made during the implementation process.

The third section presents the evaluation data. It starts by explaining the methods adopted for evaluation, followed by results and discussion.

The conclusion section summarizes and discusses key points and elaborates on the transferability of the implementation case.

Suggestions on additional resources are offered for those interested in expanding their knowledge or perfecting TBL implementation. Key terms are succinctly defined in a final section.

BACKGROUND

Development of TBL

In the late 1970s Larry K. Michaelsen, who taught small classes at Oklahoma University Business School, was faced with the challenge of teaching a class of 120 students. Instead of turning to lectures, Dr. Michaelsen split the class into small groups and introduced sequential activities that covered the course content and required students to apply their knowledge to problems and engage in discussions. By the end of the term, Michaelsen found that most students took responsibility for their own learning and accomplished good learning outcomes; interestingly, the large class size was regarded as more conducive to learning. The instructional method, called Team-Based Learning (TBL), was refined by Michaelsen over the years and disseminated in academia (Fatmi, Hartling, Hillier, Campbell, & Oswald, 2013; Krug et al., 2016).

At the end of the 1990s, Boyd Richard and colleagues at the Baylor School of Medicine in Texas piloted TBL. In 2001 the group received funding from the US government to introduce this instructional strategy and promote TBL in health professions education. Their work, which included faculty development workshops and symposia, led to TBL implementation in many educational programs in the US and abroad. Moreover, it resulted in the establishment of TBL collaborative, a mostly higher education consortium in TBL with initiatives to promote and strengthen this instructional strategy; their website is presented in the additional resources section (Krug et al., 2016; Parmelee, Michaelsen, Cook, & Hudes, 2012)

In 2008 Michaelsen published a seminal book on TBL for the health professions education, suggested as additional reading in this chapter.

The growing interest in this instructional strategy is illustrated by an upward trend in PubMed indexed articles. A search using the term 'team-based learning' restricted to the title showed an exponential increase in indexed articles, from one in 1996 to 36 in 2019, peaking at 45 in 2017.

In a systematic review of the published literature on TBL in health professions education, the pharmacy was the second most common field of study, surpassed only by medicine. Across the different fields of study, TBL has been used at an undergraduate and postgraduate level (Reimschisel, Herring, Huang, & Minor, 2017).

In pharmacy education, TBL has been chosen for a variety of topics, in both experiments and theory-oriented modules (Lang et al., 2019; Reimschisel et al., 2017). Its use as an instructional strategy for pharmacy law and ethics has also been detailed in the literature (Hasan, 2011).

Description of the Instructional Strategy

TBL is an active learning strategy based on sequential activities: individual preparation, teamwork, and feedback.

It can comprise the main instructional strategy of a module or curriculum, replacing lectures, or complement lectures within a module. It lends itself to be used with large or small classes. For example, about 10% of the TBL studies included by Reimschisel et al. (2017) involved 400 or more studies; roughly 15% involved between 11 and 50 students.

In practice, for students, TBL is comprised of three sequential phases, depicted in Figure 1. The phases shadowed in blue are typically graded. The next sections describe the TBL phases, based on (Bollela, Senger, Tourinho, & Amaral, 2014; Krug et al., 2016; Michaelsen, 2002; Parmelee et al., 2012) unless otherwise indicated.

Figure 1. Sequential TBL stages and associated steps in each macro-unity from the students' perspective

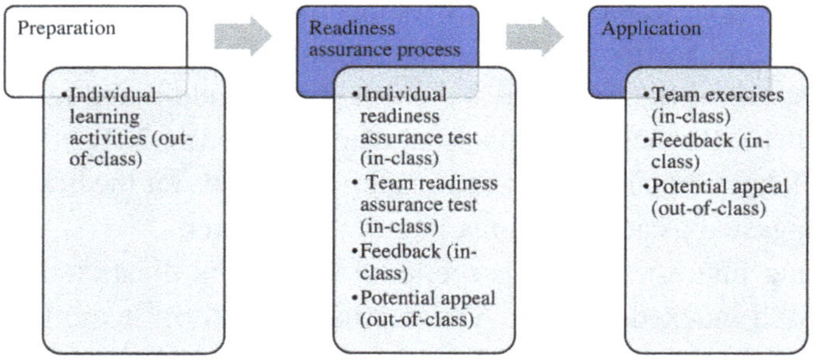

Preparation

The first phase consists of preparation. Students should engage in out-of-class learning activities, directed by a set of learning goals. While this phase is meant to be individual, and that is regarded as a facilitator by some students, others prefer to create a study group or to use the class team as a study group. ~

As a student quote by Parmelee et al. (2012) put it *Our team does not meet outside of class to prepare, but some do. It's nice that a team does not have to meet outside of class since that can be such a hassle.*

Not being prescriptive on how students should prepare and letting them figure out what works best is recommended by TBL experts.

Learning activities may include readings, videos, labs, tutorials or lectures. Two studies on students' engagement with the module content found that students preferred to have narration with their learning materials, such as recorded lectures or narrated PowerPoint slides (Reimschisel et al., 2017).

This stage provides background knowledge on the theme and forms the basis of the next TBL phase, which takes place in the classroom.

Readiness Assurance Process

The second phase encompasses individual and team readiness assurance tests (IRAT and TRAT, respectively), followed by instructor feedback. It takes place in class. The overall duration described in the literature for these in-class activities varies from 30 to 75 minutes.

IRAT and TRAT consist of the same multiple-choice questions (MCQs), aligned with the content of the preparation assignment and focusing on concepts needed to solve application problems, in the next phase.

Firstly, students complete individually a set of 10–20 of MCQs and hand the test back to the instructor. Then, students take the same test in teams. This process involves presenting and justifying individual answers and seeking consensus. Immediate feedback should be provided on whether the correct answers were selected. This can be operationalized via a template sheet covered with peeled off tags or scraping material, where the correct answer appears with a mark, such as a star. If the correct answer was not chosen, the team can discuss again and decide on another answer option, by removing an additional tag or scraping it. The teams' score decreases as more answering attempts are made. Immediate is credited with several advantages:

- Fostering team cohesion, as the "scratch-and-reveal" moment tends to engage all team members and energize them when the correct option was selected.
- Motivating discussion, as the team can immediately explore the reasons underlying the incorrect choice and get partial credit for further attempts.
- Regulating individual contributions, by instilling caution in dominant members, who pushed towards a non-consensual option that proved wrong, and by empowering passive members, unable to defend correct choices that would have helped the team getting the right answer. Peers have a role in this process, as they will tend to explore answer options from other members or to encourage the participation of members who usually "go with the flow".

Globally, the TRAT process favors knowledge construction by raising awareness of potentially unsettled learning issues through group discussion. Students' commitment to the preparation phase is critical to effectively contribute to knowledge construction and decision-making. From the interpersonal skills perspective, this process encourages the development of communication and negotiation skills.

Another form of feedback is a clarification by a content-expert instructor. This takes place when teams have completed the test and the instructor surveys the global answers to each question. This allows each team to compare their choices with those of others; additionally, it creates an opportunity for airing doubts and reasoning about choices, promoting a better understanding of concepts. When the immediate feedback assessment technique is used teams can be urged to select challenging questions for the whole class to discuss. During this process, or as a wrap-up of the session, the instructor can clarify issues that were not well understood and briefly review contents.

At the end of this phase, students should feel confident to move on to the next phase, which involves more complex problems.

An appeal can be made when a team regards an alternative answer as more correct than the one designated as 'best' by the instructor. This process happens out-of-class. Generally, the appealing team must provide, in writing, either a revised version of the MCQ and its rationale or a well-founded argument backing-up their contention. In both cases, it is expected that literature on the topic being addressed is cited and referenced. If the instructor accepts the case for changing an MCQ, the appealing team receives credit for that question; credit may be extended to individual grades (Farland et al., 2013).

Figure 2. Designing effective TBL application exercises

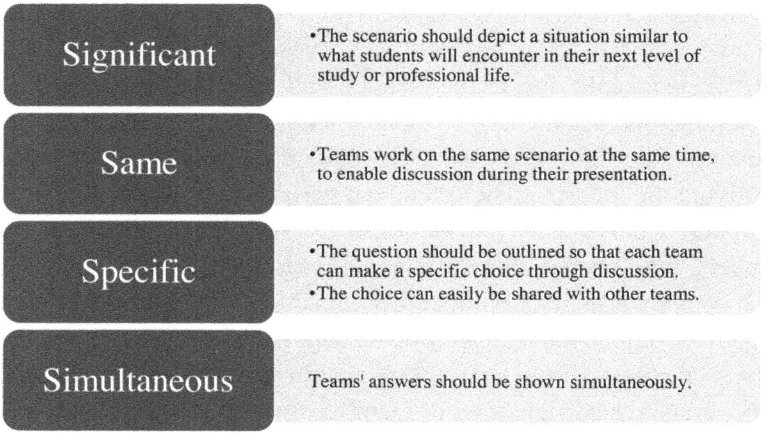

The appeal process has several advantages. Firstly, it provides an opportunity to revisit learning materials and training critical thinking and reasoning. Secondly, it nurtures a sense of fairness and helps instructors fine-tuning MCQs. Finally, it avoids diversion during class by students dwelling on their dissatisfaction with a particular MCQ; the appeal enables these students to reflect on their position and to challenge the question and answer options in a more constructive fashion.

Team Application

This phase is regarded as the most important for knowledge consolidation; the literature suggests that, overall, it can last between one and four hours.

It involves in-class exercises that allow students to apply concepts learned previously. Exercises should challenge students, through teamwork, to make interpretations, evaluations, and synthesize information, culminating in the choice of an MCQ answer. A few sequential steps are involved. Firstly, students are given an initial exercise; after answering the teams come together to present and discuss their work, explaining their rationale if requested, in a process facilitated by the instructor. Then another exercise is presented, and the steps are repeated.

The '4S' principle is recommended to formulate effective exercises; 4S' stands for 'Significant', 'Same', 'Specific' and 'Simultaneous' (Figure 2).

'Significant' exercises should come with enough detail for interpretation but should not overwhelm students. Answers should only be achieved through critical thinking, in-depth discussion, and debate within the team; they should not be readily available in sources such as textbooks or websites.

Although teams oversee answering the 'Same' exercises, ideally different teams will select different options for answers, to stimulate inter-team debate.

'Specific' exercises mean that teams should not be asked to produce long documents, which tends to result in work division as opposed to stimulating intra-team discussion.

'Simultaneous' answers promote accountability for reaching and defending decisions, allow immediate feedback and encourage discussion between the teams. Calling for volunteers or selecting randomly a team to give their answer reduces students' motivation to get the right answer, if they are not reporting can always defer to the team who reported first, by either agreeing or saying they did not have the time to reach an agreement (Parmelee et al., 2012).

Out-of-class appeals are encouraged, as described in the readiness assurance process.

Planning TBL

Unsurprisingly, Michaelsen (2002) regards the cohesiveness of student learning groups as a key factor, which, in turn, results in other positive outcomes of team-based learning.

Turning a small group into a cohesive learning team depends on four essential principles (Table 1); these inform the steps and activities entailed in TBL, both for students and instructors.

Table 1. Four essential principles of team-based learning according to Michaelsen (2002)

1. Groups must be properly formed and managed.
2. Students must be made accountable for their individual and group work.
3. Group assignments must promote both learning and team development.
4. Students must have frequent and timely feedback.

Whilst the former section described the instructional strategy from the students' perspective, this section focuses on the instructor's activities.

Organizing the Module

The first step is dividing the course content into the macro-units of instruction. Typically, each module contains four to seven macro-units, based on major topics. Michaelsen (2002) suggests that each macro-unit of instruction corresponds to 2 to 4 textbook chapters and/or other readings related to the theme.

Nonetheless, teaching and learning activities are not considered the best starting point; they should be selected after setting learning objectives and defining feedback and assessment activities.

This framework, called backward design, was put forward by Wiggins and Jay McTighe in 1998 for designing courses and content units (Bowen, 2017). Backward design is credited with several benefits, such as centering lessons in the desired outputs (not on the books and activities teachers are comfortable with), as well as promoting transparency and intentionality (activities have a purpose aligned with learning objectives). In adapting the backward design to TBL, Parmelee et al. (2012) stress that situational factors, as students' prior knowledge and the course year, should be considered.

The most important learning objectives in TBL are the "doing objectives", i.e. defining what students will do with the acquired knowledge. Instructors can set these objectives by asking themselves "'What do I want my students to be able to do at the end of the session that they could not do before?'' (Michaelsen, 2002; Parmelee et al., 2012). Other learning objectives focus on concepts students must know in order to achieve the "doing objectives". To avoid unnecessary minutiae in "concept objectives" Wiggins and McTighe (1998) suggest prioritizing content based on three questions (Table 2). Information regarding enduring understandings can be adapted to derive learning objectives.

Learning objectives should be worded using action verbs (e.g. identify, list, explain, calculate, compare, analyze).

Table 2. Wiggins and McTighe process for establishing curricular priorities

1. What should participants hear, read, view, explore or otherwise encounter?	• Knowledge worth being familiar with • Lowest priority content
2. What knowledge and skills should participants master?	• Important to know and do • Information students should know when they leave the course.
3. What are big ideas and important understandings participants should retain?	• Enduring understandings • Information students should remember when they complete the course • Highest priority content

(cited by Bowen, 2017)

Once learning objectives have been set, the feedback and assessment activities should be defined. In TBL the latter consists of team application exercises and, working backward, related readiness assurance tests. As previously mentioned, one form of feedback is a clarification by the instructor when teams have completed the assessments.

A review should be organized by the instructor *ab initio*, after creating the team application and readiness assurance questions. A well-designed clarification review encompasses content that will predictably emerge as challenging in the TRAT discussions; it is neither a lecture nor a comprehensive review of all concepts. Its purpose is to aid preparation for the team application exercises (Parmelee et al., 2012).

Finally, preparation activities (e.g. readings, videos, lectures) aligned with the assessment and the learning objectives should be prepared.

Securing the Right Infrastructure

The ideal classrooms for TBL are those enabling students to seat in small circles or around tables tailored to team sizes. Seating a five to seven-member team around a table for people curtails the closeness necessary for teamwork.

The ideal classroom allows instructors to see all students and students to students to see each other. During feedback and discussion students should also be able to hear each other without an amplification system; if an amplification system is needed microphones should ideally be placed in each table or cluster area. Passing around a single microphone is deemed as unpractical (Parmelee et al., 2012)

Forming Groups

In work and learning contexts, groups and teams have similarities, namely being comprised of two or more people who interact to deliver an output. It is commonly accepted, however, that differences exist between a group and a team.

A key difference is that team members have a mutual understanding of each other's strengths and weaknesses and can work synergic, achieving much more together than individual members would. Contrarily to groups, in which each member is responsible for their work, work outputs in teams are produced collectively. Figure 3 summarizes strategies to form groups that will evolve into a cohesive learning team.

Figure 3. Strategies to promote cohesive learning teams
Source: based on Michaelsen (2002)

Minimizing barriers to group cohesiveness	Distributing member resources	Ensuring diversity	Safeguarding group permanency
• Existing relationship between a subset of members (e.g. boyfriend/girlfriend, fraternity brothers) • Existing subgroup based on background factors such as nationality, culture or native language	• Distribute assets (e.g. work experience, academic performance) • Distribute liabilities (negative attitudes towards the course, limited fluency in the language in which the module is conducted)	• Groups must be as heterogenous as possible in regard to characteristics pertinent to team formation	• Groups should stay together as long as possible (e.g. a semester or an academic year)

It is not wise to let students form groups; not only they do not possess the information required to assure balanced and diverse groups, but they also tend to select friends or colleagues with whom they have a good relationship, creating barriers to group cohesiveness. It should, therefore, be the instructor's responsibility to form groups.

Operationalizing the strategies depicted in Figure 4 requires data gathering about students' characteristics that could potentially impact the group's success. This can be done before the first class, by inquiring the teaching staff. Defining key characteristics is strongly influenced by context; it can include students' background (rural versus urban), nationality and resources available (e.g. laptop). Gender diversity is also desired.

Classifying learning styles, via, for instance, Kolb Learning Style Inventory and VARK (Visual, Aural, Read/Write Kinesthetic) questionnaire, or personality typologies, through Myers Briggs Type Indicator or Keirsey Temperament Sorter, has been advocated (Farland et al., 2013; Krug et al., 2016). Once data have been gathered, assigning students to groups warrants a decision on group size. Group size should enable resources to adequality respond to challenging tasks without preventing full participation of all members. The recommended size for ideal team development is five to seven members (Michaelsen, 2002; Parmelee et al., 2012). The instructor can then determine the total number of groups, based on group size and the size of the class. Finally, students can be distributed across groups according to their characteristics.

Safeguarding group permanency recognizes that groups evolve into effectively functioning teams; when groups are reformed the development process restarts from the beginning. For example, in newly formed groups disagreement or confronting opinions may be perceived as uncomfortable, therefore it is not unusual to make decisions by voting. In this stage, groups are inclined to rely on their most competent member. As joint work evolves, groups have generally learned to deal with disagreement or conflicts and realize that it is more effective to cater resources from all members, by voicing different perspectives first, discuss them and then come to a consensus.

Underlining the importance of permanent groups is unsurprising considering the literature on group developmental processes in other, non-learning contexts. Most authors posit that groups go through several development phases if allowed to exist over an extended period; the "forming, storming, norming and performing" is probably the most influential model on the topic. It argues that groups evolve through different stages until a performing stage is achieved, in which *roles become flexible and functional, and group energy is channeled into the task. Structural issues have been resolved, and structure can now become supportive of task performance* (Tuckman, 1965). As in other contexts, changing learning groups during the development phase disrupts their progress into effective teams.

Creating groups in the presence of students, commonly in the first class, offers an opportunity to explain the rationale for the process and to collect data on students' characteristics, otherwise unavailable, through verbal questioning (e.g. "Which town are you from?"; "How many of you have work experience?") or instruments (e.g. learning styles or personality questionnaires). A variant of this process is observing the dynamics of provisionally formed diverse groups in the first class and then forming definite groups in the second class (Krug et al., 2016).

While group formation can be completed in the first class, it requires prior consideration and therefore is presented in the planning section.

Grading

The existence of an assessment system promoting engagement in learning and group interaction is regarded as essential. Therefore, grading should account for both individual and group performance. As for other instructional strategies resorting to small group work, there is a concern of rewarding fairly members' contributions.

A way to tackle this concern is employing also peer evaluation (Michaelsen, 2002). Including a qualitative component in peer evaluation trains students in giving and receiving constructive feedback from peers, which is valuable in a learning context and their future professional lives (Parmelee et al., 2012). Peer evaluation is also credited to accelerate progress through the stages of team formation (Farland et al., 2013).

Peer evaluation involves collecting data from students regarding each of his/her teammates' contribution to the team's performance and their learning, and then making the information available to individual students in an aggregated format, without identifying who provide it.

The quantitative component of peer evaluation consists of a numerical assessment of each student. This can be implemented, for instance, by asking each student to anonymously divide 100 points for team members based on their individual contribution; scores are then compiled and fed into the grading scheme in an appropriate format.

The qualitative component consists of students' comments regarding each of his/her teammates' contributions. Providing constructive feedback is challenging for most people. It is worthy aiding students in this process through simple guidelines, that promote comments on existing positive behaviors and their improvement; this helps them adjusting behavior without causing discomfort or resentment. In writing, this can be operationalized by asking students ''What is the single most valuable 'contribution' this person makes to your team?'' and ''What is the single most important 'thing' this person could do to more effectively help your team?'' (Parmelee et al., 2012).

Ultimately, students should be reminded that feedback is about offering information *with the intention of narrowing the gap between actual and desired performance*(Cantillon & Sargeant, 2008); it involves judgments about people's performance, not their personal traits.

The process of compiling and feeding back results to students, both qualitative and quantitative, can be streamlined via available software; some educators will also grade the qualitative component of peer evaluation (Krug et al., 2016).

One important issue is how often peer evaluation is conducted. Planning this issue should consider the amount of time students have spent as a team; working together for a few hours will predictably result in low levels of cohesiveness and perhaps well-founded opinions. Studies on TBL in pharmacy education reported conducting peer evaluation once or twice during the semester. Numerous evaluations are reputed to cause "survey fatigue" and disturb team development by reinforcing the dominant element(s) (Farland et al., 2013).

While peer evaluation generally takes place out-of-class, team members can be encouraged to provide feedback directly to one another in class.

The literature provided examples of TBL grading schemes (Parmelee et al., 2012), such as:

- IRAT: 25%.
- TRAT: 35%.
- Team application: 35%.
- Peer evaluation: 5%.

It is suggested that students should be involved in determining the weight of each component, within limits set by the instructor (Michaelsen, 2002; Parmelee et al., 2012); this can be achieved through a group exercise in the first class.

Finally, the weight of TBL grading in the final module grade should reflect the proportion of time devoted to this instructional strategy. For instance, in the 12-week module where TBL is employed for approximately half of the contact hours, it should count for about 50% of the final grade (Parmelee et al., 2012).

Implementing TBL

First-Class

TBL is different from instructional strategies that students are typically familiar with. Therefore, the first class should be used to explain how this instructional strategy works and its rationale, in addition to other important points (Table 3).

One of the suggested activities is comparing a TBL module with a traditional module, focusing on how the learning objectives are accomplished (Michaelsen, 2002). Another possible activity is, once groups are set, in-class demonstration of the readiness assurance process, resorting to the module syllabus or an article about TBL as the "content" material (Michaelsen, 2002; Parmelee et al., 2012).

Ideally, these materials will be covered in advance, to illustrate the need for preparing for class. If unfeasible, students can be given time in class to read the materials. Going through the IRAT, TRAT and subsequent feedback and discussion promotes an understanding of the process and may reduce anxiety associated with the first readiness assurance tests, which are normally graded. Parmelee et al. (2012) recommend that the exercise is taken a stage further, by conducting team application.

Table 3. Key instructor activities in the first class

• *Explaining how TBL works and why is being used.*
• *Completing group formation.*
• *Clarifying the grading system.*

(Michaelsen, 2002)

Managing Classes

The section describing TBL highlighted the role of the instructor, as content-expert, in providing feedback, addressing knowledge gaps and misconceptions, summarizing key issues and, ultimately, in aiding students to achieve the learning objectives.

Facilitating TBL classes demands also communication and organizational skills, that will be detailed in turn.

Communication skills are required to develop and maintain an open and interactive environment in the classroom (Farland et al., 2013). Within communication, facilitation skills are crucial to fully unravel TBL potential. Levine et al. (2019) developed the facilitator instrument for team-based learning (FIT), designed to assess TBL facilitation. The instrument was piloted with almost 3000 students in seven North American medical schools, it showed adequate psychometric properties. Its 11 items (Table 4) can be used as a checklist by instructors employing TBL.

Table 4. Checklist for TBL instructors derived from the 11-item FIT

1. Actively listens to students' responses.
2. Clarifies concepts when they are initially confusing.
3. Elicits discussion of alternative answers.
4. Responds to questions with thought
5. Prompts learners to support opinions with evidence.
6. Redirects nonproductive discussions.
7. Concludes team discussions in a way that makes the key principles clear.
8. Helps students understand the significance of the issues discussed.
9. Highlights the most important points of the session.
10. Tries to engage all teams during discussions.
11. Uses questions to deepen students' thinking.

(Levine et al., 2019)

For instance, questions to deepen students' thinking may include "Why did your team choose this option?", "Explain your thoughts when choosing this option", "Tell me about your rationale, why do you think it is better than the one we just heard?". Getting reports from all the groups may be tedious, particularly if there are many teams in the classroom; it suffices to debate the answers from a couple of teams with different answers and then asking the class if there are doubts or questions.

Organizational skills include monitoring group work by walking around the classroom, managing time and moderating the answers.

Walking around the room serves the purpose of listening to the teams' conversations, understanding how they are processing the assignment and use it in the discussions (Parmelee et al., 2012).

Managing time in each assignment can be done by explicitly stating the allocated time and by issuing countdown warnings (Farland et al., 2013). For instance, when the assignment starts the instructor tells students they have 10 minutes to complete it and writes on the board the starting and finishing time. Halfway down the line, students get a first warning (5 minutes left); a final warning is made when 1 minute is left. When the time limit is reached the instructor can grab the entire class's attention by asking teams who need more time to raise their hands. If needed, teams can be allowed one or two more minutes to finish, if not the instructor can move on to survey the answers.

To improve students' accountability the instructor should select students by name when moderating the answers, preferably with a system that ensures equity of participation. Mobile applications are available to assist in this process (see additional resources). Simultaneous answers in team application exercises can be operationalized by showing numbered or letter cards to the whole class, through audience response systems or by sticking the answers on the classroom walls. The latter allows teams to place notes on the answers of others for further discussion.

Evidence on the Impact of TBL in Pharmacy and Other Health Disciplines

Several systematic reviews have been published on the impact of TBL in pharmacy and health professions education (Fatmi et al., 2013; Lang et al., 2019; Reimschisel et al., 2017).

Fatmi and colleagues included 14 studies in their review, encompassing over 3500 participants. Only one study had a randomized controlled design; the others were classified by the authors as non-randomized controlled trials (2), prospective cohort studies (2), retrospective cohort study (1), concurrent cohort study (1) and non-concurrent cohorts (7).

All 14 studies assessed knowledge as a learning outcome; seven also assessed learner reaction. Out of 14 studies, 7 yielded a significant increase in knowledge scores for the TBL group (four reported no difference and three showed improvement with uncertain statistical significance). Only one study showed a significant improvement in learner reaction for the TBL group, indicating mixed reactions to this instructional strategy (Fatmi et al., 2013).

Reimschisel et al. (2017) summarized the published literature employing the TBL conceptual framework proposed by Michaelsen, which encompasses seven components: design elements, teacher and learner attitudes, contextual factors, team characteristics, learners' engagement with course content, a pattern of member engagement within teams and learning outcomes. A total of 118 articles were included in this systematic review. The most frequently researched framework component was teacher and learner attitudes (97 articles; 82%), followed by learning outcomes (85 articles; 72%).

Of these studies, 79% compared TBL learning outcomes to another instructional strategy, generally the didactic lecture. TBL had a positive effect in about two-thirds of the studies (52/85; 61%), often measured by examination or standardized tests grades. Weaker students appear to benefit more from TBL than their academically stronger counterparts.

The superiority of TBL in long-term retention, when compared to lectures or other instructional strategies, remains unproven. The authors discussed possible sources of bias and their direction: a higher level of focus from instructors on the new instructional strategy, which could favor TBL, less experienced with the newer strategy, which could disfavor TBL, and higher levels of interest from students due to the novelty, which could favor TBL (or any new instructional strategy). About a fifth of the studies assessed TBL impact after one or two sessions, which may be insufficient to fully unravel the potential of this strategy, especially in light of the time needed to form a performing team (Reimschisel et al., 2017).

The studies included in the two aforementioned reviews were mainly from the United States, which raises a concern about the generalizability of findings to education contexts in other countries. Another concern is the lack of experimental studies; while Fatmi et al. (2013) included only one randomized controlled trial (RCT) in their review, Reimschisel et al. (2017) did not provide information on the design of included studies. These concerns may be partly minimized by a recent systematic review and meta-analysis on the effect of TBL in pharmacy education in China (Lang et al., 2019). These authors demonstrated, based on 12 RCTs (total of 1271 participants, 631 in the TBL group), that TBL was more effective than traditional lectures in developing scores of objective theoretical tests. The fact that TBL helped learners in distinct geographies and cultures is encouraging to educators wishing to implement this active instructional strategy.

There is also a need of broadening the definition of learning outcomes to skills predictability improved by TBL and useful for health care professionals, but not measured in written tests, such as the ability to work in a team.

IMPLEMENTING TBL IN A PHARMACY LAW AND ETHICS MODULE

Context

The teaching of ethics and pharmacy legislation is enshrined in the syllabuses of most integrated master's degree courses in Pharmaceutical Sciences in Portugal as a required module. At the Higher Education Institution where the author lectures this was initially a year five-module (3 ECTS, 55 contact hours). As part of an overall course revision in 2014/15 the topic is currently taught in year 3 (4 ECTS, 52 contact hours).

In either case, the module aims to contribute to the acquisition of knowledge and the development of attitudes that allow future professionals to practice in accordance with ethics and the existing legal framework. The syllabus covers content related to health care ethics, professional norms and legislation related to medicines, community pharmacy, non-prescription medicines outlets, and medical devices.

Typically, class size varies between 25 and 30 students and there is a single instructor (the author). Although some students may enroll in elective practice internships, mostly during summer periods, their contact with professional practice is generally limited to the second semester of year 5.

This creates difficulties in relating the module contents with practice and occasional lack of engagement in learning. This aspect was the main drive to implement an active learning strategy with demonstrated benefit in theoretical-practical classes, which represent roughly half of the contact hours. The author firstly implemented problem-based learning, which proved too resource-intensive, and was then replaced by team-based learning.

Overview of Planning and Implementation

Planning and implementation followed generally the recommendations presented in the previous section.

While major changes to the instructional strategy are discouraged, as they may compromise its effectiveness (Parmelee et al., 2012), minor adaptations in light of context particularities are arguably inevitable.

This section details key aspects of planning and implementation concerning a pharmacy law and ethics module.

The process started in the academic year 2015/16. Content covered in theoretical-practical classes, two hours each, was split into six macro-units of instruction. These have suffered slight changes over the years.

The approach took by the author for each macro-unit is probably best described as "iterative design" (Figure 4). Planned learning objectives, assessment activities, and preparation activities were compared and contrasted in loops until the author was satisfied with the meaningfulness of learning objectives and its alignment with the remaining elements.

Consideration was given to the workload estimated for the preparation in relation to the time available for autonomous work. As a rule of thumb, students spend more time in these advanced assignments than the author anticipates.

Figure 4. Iterative design for each macro-unit of instruction

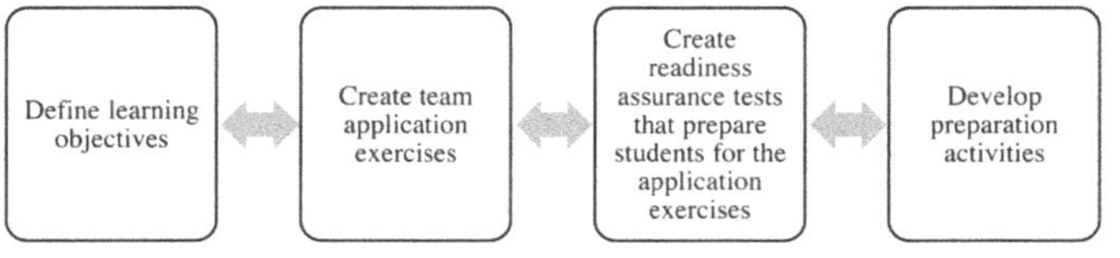

A clarification review was prepared for some units through Microsoft Office PowerPoint slides.

Planning included liaising with the Institution's academic office to secure the best possible infrastructure. While fixed seating auditoriums have been suggested as a possibility (Parmelee et al., 2012), the author's experience is that they are not functional.

Classroom size is also important. The author's experience is that classrooms too small result in excessive clustering of students, inter-team inputs and sometimes a perception by teams of disrupting noise levels. While noise in the room is acknowledged as a TBL feature indicating healthy group dynamics (Parmelee et al., 2012), it requires management when it interferes with students' learning experience.

In the initial year of implementation, when multiple issues necessitated attention, groups were formed by a random selection of students. The author realized this led to an uneven distribution of resources (e.g. clustering Erasmus students in one group) and lack of diversity (e.g. no gender balance). The process was perfected by looking at the list of enrolled students prior to each class and creating provisional groups based on key characteristics (e.g. age, gender, students with worker status). Groups were then fine-tuned in class following data gathering about additional characteristics.

The author has experience in using the Honey-Alonso questionnaire of Learning Styles to form groups, but its application was deemed unpractical to fit in the first class, mainly due to time management issues. In terms of group size, the author's experience corroborates the importance of forming groups of no less than five students. Evidence on group size shows most positive experiences and better performance in four to seven members' groups (Farland et al., 2013); however, groups of four members may become critically deprived of resources should one member miss the class.

Several authors suggest that groups must work together for at least 40 hours to allow the formation of performing teams (Farland et al., 2013; Krug et al., 2016). This will be contingent on the contact hours of the module and often not amenable to change by educators. The author ensured group permanency throughout the semester and remained conscious of the pertinence of other strategies to promote cohesive learning teams (Figure 4).

The grading of the Pharmacy Law and Ethics module and the weight of TBL are depicted in Figure 5. Involving students in determining the weight of each TBL component was unfeasible, as the module syllabus, which includes grading schemes, must receive Institutional approval prior to the semester beginning. The lowest grade in each test (IRATs, TRATs and application exercises) has been discarded since the first year of implementation. This can account for students' absences due to unforeseen events and suboptimal preparation, which tends to occur towards the end of the semester when students have multiple assignments.

Peer evaluation has not been implemented yet. The reasons are two-fold. Firstly, students resisted the idea, which is unsurprising (Farland et al., 2013; Reimschisel et al., 2017). By way of illustration, in previous studies students have made negative remarks about peer evaluation or completed it in a meaningless way, by attributing the same rating to all team members.

Figure 5. The overall grading of the Pharmacy Law and Ethics module (2015/16)

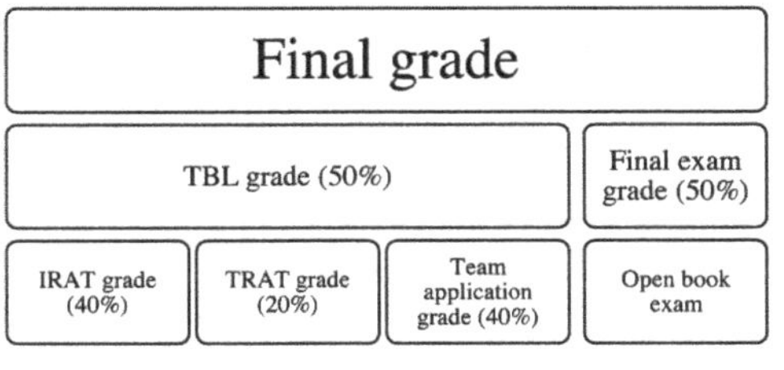

Table 5 details the operationalization of the sequential TBL stages and associated steps. Initially, all readiness assurance tests were paper-based. The author has not found "scratch-and-reveal" forms in Portugal and chose to deploy traditional pen-and-paper formats, which do not allow immediate feedback. In the first two academic years of implementation partial credit was allowed in IRATs by allowing students to distribute four points across the four MCQ answer options (Bollela et al., 2014; Farland et al., 2013).

However, the author became reluctant about this approach, in particular for IRATs. Distributing points between answer options may reward team discussion in TRATs where teams are not confident of their choices; in IRATs may encourage the undesirable behavior of placing one point on each answer choice due to lack of preparation and get some credit.

In the academic year of 2017/18, paperless IRATs were implemented using the Moodle learning management system. Online Moodle tests have convenient features to support TRATs, such as enabling multiple attempts for answering with partial credit. The downside, which has hampered its use, is the fact that students will contact MCQs in an environment with little invigilation. Under these circumstances the possibility of unduly copying MCQs (by screen captures, for example) must be considered; managing this situation may require the writing-up of new MCQs every year, which is challenging. The author has noticed that her estimations of the difficulty level of MCQs are sometimes not accurate; this may produce questions too easy to stimulate debate during the TRAT.

Significance in team application exercises was ensured by resorting to real-life cases involving pharmacists, either from the author's experience or from media accounts (e.g. "Pharmacy Permitted Man to View Video of Wife Purchasing Pregnancy Test" or "Pharmacy error leads to fatal medication mix-up"). Open-ended questions were deployed, mainly due to the recognition of the importance of open-ended problem solving; this variation has been acknowledged by others (Farland et al., 2013).

Simultaneous reporting was accomplished by seating a rapporteur from each group in the front of the classroom, in a semi-circle. Each student reads their group's answer; once all have finished the instructor leads the discussion. As for TRATs, students can select who speaks for the group in a rotation system, in which all members must function as rapporteurs.

The turn-around time for appeals, which are based on a form developed for this purpose, is kept brief by allowing one week for teams to submit them and one week for the author to respond. Appeals have seldom been used by teams during the 4-year implementation period.

Table 5. Operationalization of TBL in each unit of instruction of the pharmacy law and ethics module

Phase	Timing	Place	Process	Modality	Duration
Preparation	Week 0	Out-of-class	One-page preparation sheet (list of learning objectives + description of the learning activities + copies or references of the learning resources – e.g. book chapter, legal acts)	Digital (Moodle)	The time necessary for engaging in the learning activities
Readiness assurance process	Week 1	In-class	IRAT (10 MCQs)	Digital (Moodle)	10 minutes
		In-class	TRAT (10 MCQs, identical to the IRAT)	Paper-based	20 – 30 minutes
			Instructor feedback	Face-to-face discussion	45 – 60 minutes
			Clarification review by the instructor	PowerPoint presentation	5 -10 minutes
	By the end of week 2	Out-of-class	Potential appeal	Digital (email)	The time necessary for producing the written appeal
Team application	Week 2	In-class	4 short open-ended questions on one real-world scenario, presented in turn	Paper-based	15 minutes per question
			Simultaneous presentation of answers, discussion, and feedback	Face-to-face discussion	10 minutes per question
	By the end of week 3		Potential appeal	Digital (email)	The time necessary for producing the written appeal

EVALUATING TBL IN A PHARMACY LAW AND ETHICS MODULE

Participants and Procedure

The population consisted of students from the pharmacy law and ethics module in the academic year 2015/2016. An anonymous and online monitoring questionnaire was launched at the end of the first semester (3 ECTS module) and the second semester

(4 ECTS module, new curriculum), complementary to Institutional assessment regularly performed.

The on-line questionnaire included six closed questions on TBL with a three-point answer scale (positive, negative, undecided) and an open-ended question.

Numerical data were subjected to descriptive statistics with the help of SPSS version 24. Textual data from the open question were thematically coded.

Results and Discussion

A total of 43 and 17 questionnaires were obtained, corresponding to the first and second semesters, yielding a response rate of 49% and 71%, respectively. The results in both modules were broadly similar, so data were analyzed together. One student objected to the use of his/her data for scientific purposes; this questionnaire was subsequently excluded. Fifty-nine questionnaires were considered for analysis.

The sample was comprised mainly of female students (47; 79.7%), with an average age of 22.8 years (minimum 20; maximum 28). About one-fifth of the respondents had worker status (11; 18.6%).

Students had a largely positive perspective on TBL concerning the motivation for working out-of-class, learning, and relationship with the group (Figure 7). The two additional questions on TBL confirmed this positive perspective, as most students (53; 89.8%) stated that if they could choose, they would opt for TBL as the instructional strategy to use in the theoretical-practical classes. About 9 out of 10 students would recommend TBL to peers (52, 88.1%).

Figure 6. Students' perspectives on TBL (2015/16; n=59)

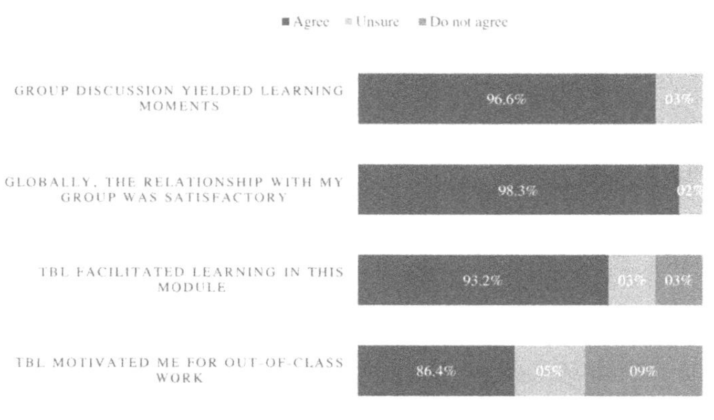

Six students answered the open question. The comments were categorized as "appreciation of the instructional strategy" (e.g. "allows us to learn, unlike the other modules, where we have to memorize things that vanish the day after the exam") and "suggestions" (e.g. "more objective MCQs, less workload").

Undoubtedly, surveyed students had a favorable reaction to TBL; this is in accordance with informal feedback obtained throughout the semester. Taken together with the response rates, it may be reasonable to assume that the results are generalizable to the entire student population.

In the literature, students' reactions to TBL are not unanimous (Fatmi et al., 2013; Reimschisel et al., 2017). While some studies report positive feedback, others found, for example, that students preferred lectures over TBL (Reimschisel et al., 2017). One possible explanation for the overwhelming preference for TBL in the pharmacy law and ethics module is the fact that lectures would not have been an option for theoretical-practical classes, in which active instructional strategies are generally pursued. The author's experience of changing from traditional lectures to "flipped classroom" in another module suggests this encounters more resistance from students, which is not unexpected (Rotellar & Cain, 2016).

One of the students' comments highlighted the issue of the workload associated with TBL. Fatmi et al. (2013) urges educators to take actions to minimize potentially negative students' reactions and have hypothesized that the increased workload may be one of the reasons justifying dissatisfaction. In the pharmacy law and ethics, the workload issue has been addressed by reducing the six initial macro-units to five; in-class time released is used at the end of the semester for recapping contents.

As expected, students acknowledged the existence of peer teaching and learning. Whilst the results indicate that group work was mostly satisfactory, there is little data on team development, that could be obtained from peer evaluation or the analysis of IRATs and TRATs scores. For example, Michaelsen (2002) consistently found that 99% of the teams outperform their best member. By the end of the term, he shares with students an analysis of five IRATs and TRATs scores for each team, which invariably illustrates this pattern, to facilitate learning about the value of teams.

Another drawback of the current evaluation is the fact that a non-validated questionnaire was used. The Team-Based Learning Student Assessment Instrument (TBL-SAI), comprised of 33 items across three subscales - accountability, preference for a lecture or team-based learning, and student satisfaction - has demonstrated to be valid and reliable when used with North-American nursing students (Mennenga, 2012). More recently, this instrument showed adequate psychometric properties in a sample of pharmacy students in two British Schools (Nation, Tweddell, & Rutter, 2016). To the author's best knowledge there is no Portuguese version of TBL-SAI; rigorous translation and validation of this instrument to the Portuguese reality requires resources beyond the regular pedagogical monitoring, which may comprise future research work.

CONCLUSION

TBL is an active learning strategy based on individual and team activities, conducted out and in-class. It represents a substantial change in the role of students and instructors. Students are required to take responsibility for the initial preparation of content; instructors move from imparting knowledge only to managing the overall instructional process.

This chapter offers an overview of TBL components, and on planning and implementing this instructional strategy. An account of its application in a pharmacy law and ethics module corroborates the notion that TBL is valuable across a wide range of topics and offers inspiration to those wishing to implement it in their own teaching.

The author's account on implementation also confirms that the instructor's motivation and commitment to improving teaching and learning can overcome existing obstacles. For instance, receiving training on TBL prior to implementation is advocated, either by attending a workshop or getting orientation by fellow instructors (Parmelee et al., 2012). Another suggestion is identifying a person experienced with TBL to serve as a consultant (Parmelee et al., 2012). These suggestions, which will contribute to a smoother and more efficient implementing process, both for students and instructors, maybe unattainable in countries with scarce educational support for TBL instructors. Attentive reading about TBL before implementation and careful reflection on the process implemented may suffice, without disregarding training opportunities that can meanwhile appear.

Modules using a single instructor, as the one reported in this chapter, facilitate consistency across classes. However, single instructors will not be supported by a teaching team in the peer review of questions and airing of problems and doubts, which can create difficulties.

The author's reaction to TBL accords with earlier observations, which demonstrated that instructors found it satisfying despite the additional workload, especially in the beginning. It is unquestionable that implementing TBL, globally or partly in a module or a course, has a steep launch. This workload may be managed by a stepwise approach and through digital technology.

Adopting a stepwise approach is exemplified by the gradual conversion of content into macro-units of instruction in a module or by establishing pilot TBL modules within a course; it does not mean using "bits and pieces" of the instructional strategy, which can compromise its effectiveness.

This chapter illustrated the use of digital technology support to implement TBL, mainly in the form of learning management systems for sharing information and automated grading of IRATs. The literature mentions other possibilities, which have been detailed throughout the chapter and listed in the additional resources section. Digital technology does not necessarily streamline processes; it may be costly and requires spending time to master. Instructors should carefully assess whether digital solutions are suited to their needs.

Students expressed a positive perspective about TBL as an instructional strategy for supplementing lectures in a pharmacy law and ethics module. Evaluation from a subsequent academic year remained overall positive. These perspectives, together with other favorable indicators, led to TBL maintenance until the current days.

The author is cognizant of the importance of students' feedback but subscribes to the opinion that the *merits of a novel teaching strategy cannot depend solely on student feedback* (Reimschisel et al., 2017). Students' evaluation of TBL in this module is seen as a means to end – signposting potential problems and contributing to improve students and the instructor experience – and not an end in itself.

ACKNOWLEDGMENT

I am grateful to all my students; what they have taught me over the last 12 years helped me become a better teacher. I am also indebted to those students who take the time to provide constructive feedback for improvement purposes.

REFERENCES

Bollela, V. R., Senger, M. H., Tourinho, F. S. V, & Amaral, E. (2014). Aprendizagem baseada em equipes: da teoria à prática. *Medicina (Ribeirão Preto), 47*(3), 293–300.

Bowen, R. S. (2017). *Understanding by Design.* Vanderbilt University Center for Teaching. Retrieved from https://cft.vanderbilt.edu/understanding-by-design/

Cantillon, P., & Sargeant, J. (2008). Giving feedback in clinical settings. *BMJ (Clinical Research Ed.), 337*(7681), 1292–1294. doi:10.1136/bmj.a1961 PMID:19001006

Farland, M. Z., Sicat, B. L., Franks, A. S., Pater, K. S., Medina, M. S., & Persky, A. M. (2013). Best Practices for Implementing Team-Based Learning in Pharmacy Education. *American Journal of Pharmaceutical Education, 77*(8), 177. Advance online publication. doi:10.5688/ajpe778177 PMID:24159218

Fatmi, M., Hartling, L., Hillier, T., Campbell, S., & Oswald, A. E. (2013). The effectiveness of team-based learning on learning outcomes in health professions education: BEME Guide No. 30. *Medical Teacher*, *35*(12), e1608–e1624. doi:10.3109/0142159X.2013.849802 PMID:24245519

Hasan, S. (2011). Teaching ethics to pharmacy students using a team-based learning approach. *Pharmacy Education*, *11*(1), 99–106.

Krug, R. de R., Vieira, M. S. M., & Maciel, M. V. de A. e, Erdmann, T. R., Vieira, F. C. de F., Koch, M. C., & Grosseman, S. (2016). O "Bê-Á-Bá" da Aprendizagem Baseada em Equipe. *Revista Brasileira de Educação Médica*, *40*(4), 602–610. doi:10.1590/1981-52712015v40n4e00452015

Lang, B., Zhang, L., Lin, Y., Han, L., Zhang, C., & Liu, Y. (2019). Team-based learning pedagogy enhances the quality of Chinese pharmacy education: A systematic review and meta-analysis. *BMC Medical Education*, *19*(1), 286. doi:10.118612909-019-1724-6 PMID:31357986

Levine, R. E., Hsieh, P., Kelly, P. A., Carchedi, L., Gibson, J., Haidet, P., ... Thompson, B. (2019). The Facilitator Instrument for Team-Based Learning (FIT). *Teaching and Learning in Medicine*, *1334*. Advance online publication. doi:10.1080/10401334.2019.1646653 PMID:31389259

Mennenga, H. (2012). Development and Psychometric Testing of the Team-Based Learning Student Assessment Instrument. *Nurse Educator*, *37*(4), 168–172. doi:10.1097/NNE.0b013e31825a87cc PMID:22688878

Michaelsen, L. K. (2002). Getting started with team-based learning. In *Team-based learning: a transformative use of small groups* (pp. 27–51). Praeger Publisher.

Nation, L. M., Tweddell, S., & Rutter, P. (2016). The applicability of a validated team-based learning student assessment instrument to assess United Kingdom pharmacy students' attitude toward team-based learning. *Journal of Educational Evaluation for Health Professions*, *13*, 30. doi:10.3352/jeehp.2016.13.30 PMID:27568493

Parmelee, D., Michaelsen, L. K., Cook, S., & Hudes, P. D. (2012). Team-based learning: A practical guide: AMEE Guide No. 65. *Medical Teacher*, *34*(5), 275–288. doi:10.3109/0142159X.2012.651179 PMID:22471941

Reimschisel, T., Herring, A. L., Huang, J., & Minor, T. J. (2017). A systematic review of the published literature on team-based learning in health professions education. *Medical Teacher*, *39*(12), 1–11. doi:10.1080/0142159X.2017.1340636 PMID:28664760

Rotellar, C., & Cain, J. (2016). Research, perspectives, and recommendations on implementing the flipped classroom. *American Journal of Pharmaceutical Education, 80*(2), 34. Advance online publication. doi:10.5688/ajpe80234 PMID:27073287

Tuckman, B. W. (1965). Developmental sequence in small groups. *Psychological Bulletin, 63*(6), 384–399. doi:10.1037/h0022100 PMID:14314073

ADDITIONAL READING

Michealsen, L. K., Parmalee, D. X., McMahon, L. L., & Revine, R. E. (Eds.). (2008). *Team-Based Learning for Health Professions Education: A Guide to Using Small Groups for Improving Learning. Sterling*. Stylus Publishing.

KEY TERMS AND DEFINITIONS

Course: Entire educational program in higher education required to complete a degree.

European Credit Transfer and Accumulation System (ECTS) Credits: Means of expressing the volume of learning in the European Union, based on the defined learning outcomes and their associated workload in higher education.

Macro-Unit of Instruction: Partition of a module content that can be tied together thematically.

Module: Unit of study in a higher education course, corresponding to several ECTS credits.

Chapter 8
Clinical Research and Regulatory Affairs:
Skills and Tools in Pharmacy Education

Maria Teresa Herdeiro
iBiMED, Medical Sciences Department, University of Aveiro, Portugal

Nélia Gouveia
NOVA Medical School, Faculdade de Ciências Médicas, Universidade NOVA de Lisboa, Portugal

Fátima Roque
Health Sciences School, Polytechnic Institute of Guarda, Portugal

ABSTRACT

Clinical research is a large umbrella, and it mainly includes the implementation of clinical studies/trials. This field is crucial to assess the value of new developments in healthcare, be it new therapeutic interventions, medical devices, or systems of care. In order to protect human rights, the implementation of clinical trials is complex and extremely costly. In this context, medicines and medical devices are strongly regulated products before and after the market authorization. So during their training, pharmacists must develop skills in the area of regulatory affairs, design and methodology of clinical trials, and other clinical studies, as well as in the management of clinical projects to be prepared for the challenges of the clinical research and market access processes. With that purpose, knowledge and skills for clinical research should be developed in association with regulatory affairs.

DOI: 10.4018/978-1-7998-4486-0.ch008

INTRODUCTION

Clinical research encompasses all investigations related to treatment, prevention, diagnosis, or prognosis of disease or improvement of health (Ioannidis, 2016). Clinical trial (CT) studies, designed to investigate the safety and the efficacy or effectiveness of a medicine, are considered one of the most appropriate methodologies that respond to such questions, consequently leading to a change in decision making (European Medicines Agency, n.d.; Ioannidis, 2016). In fact, randomized CTs (RCTs) are at the top of the pyramid of scientific evidence due to the robustness that can be achieved with this kind of study design.

To ensure both the highest standards of safety for participants and transparency of all information, CTs are strictly regulated by the European Medicines Agency (EMA) and Food and Drug Administration (FDA), respectively in Europe and the USA, and must obey specific requirements (European Medicines Agency, 2020b; Food and Drug Administration, 2020). Furthermore, the European regulation is also transposed into national law, in each country, making the process even more regulated in order to assure compliance with Good Clinical Practices (GCP).

During a CT, the changes in benefits, harms, cost, and other factors are considered before approving or not a new therapeutic intervention, medical device, or system of care. Moreover, even after the marketing authorization (MA), a clinical trial-resulting product must be constantly monitored and evaluated. The faster development and the increased complexity of regulated medicines and medical devices make the demand for ensuring the protection of both human and animal health by regulators a hard task. For this reason, the industry regulatory workforce is facing several difficulties to keep current knowledge concerning innovation and all the processes related to the regulatory science and new strategies, allowing regulators to stay in line with drugs in development, and patients to have faster access to innovative medicines (Altman et al., 2015; Philip A. Hines et al., 2019, 2020; Rasi, 2017).

These strategies must encompass the growing ecosystem of innovation in the development of human and veterinary medicines (Philip A. Hines et al., 2020).

To ensure the academic programs are following the market needs, and students are acquiring competencies derived from analysis of societal and patient needs, worldwide universities have adapted their programs by adding the regulatory science course (Moghissi et al., 2020).

The efficacy of an educational program is highly dependent on the perception of students' gaps and needs. It has been reported that pharmacy students have gaps in subjects such as communication, safety clinical research, and regulatory science (Warholak et al., 2011). Moreover, according to the literature, the process of learning includes five stages of skill acquisitions: (a) novice, (b) advanced beginner, (c) competence, (d) proficiency, and (e) expertise, during which the learner will improve their competencies (Dreyfus, 2004). In the last decades, to ameliorate the process of learning and improve pharmacist students' skills, academic institutions have been focused on finding an alternative to the traditional educational system, that is rigid and indifferent to societal and patients' demands.

The pharmacy literature defines "standard competencies" as *the skills, attitudes, values, beliefs, and other qualities, gained by individuals from education, training, and clinical experience, which enable them to practice effectively in the pharmacy profession* (Katoue & Schwinghammer, 2020).

In the last decade, the concept of "competency-based education" (CBE) has emerged. CBE aims to train the required clinical competencies that will best respond to societal healthcare needs. Frank et al.'s (Frank et al., 2010) point of view on outcome-based competencies is a good strategy for regulatory education (Drago et al., 2016). The authors argue that instead of being centered on credit hours and classroom time, regulatory science educational training should be focused on the acquisition of key competencies (Frank et al., 2010).

CBE was created to promote the competencies development of future healthcare professionals, which will be further reflected in their ability to perform the tasks precisely, make appropriate judgments and properly deal with patients and colleagues (Brown et al., 2012; Katoue & Schwinghammer, 2020).

According to Katoue and Schwinghammer (2020), since CBE is based on the development of practitioner skills to better serve the needs of the pharmacist profession, this model may ensure the preparation of competent pharmacists and reinforce the trust of society in graduate skills (Katoue & Schwinghammer, 2020). However, the adoption of this model represents a great challenge because it requires the delineation and operationalization of competencies that can sometimes be difficult to define, develop, implement, and assess, along with the collaboration of all stakeholders involved (Katoue & Schwinghammer, 2020; Koster et al., 2017).

This chapter aims to assess the teaching methodologies on regulatory affairs, CTs, and other clinical studies, as well as the management of clinical projects necessary for training future pharmacists. Additionally, discuss the implementation of different scenarios and methodologies that cultivate curiosity and develop new skills in the students, according to the needs of the market, will also be discussed.

BACKGROUND

During their academic training, pharmacy students expect to acquire skills according to their inclinations and market demands (European Pharmaceutical Students' Association, n.d.).

In this context, the pharmacy faculties/schools join forces to dynamize and improve their educational strategies. Because of the increased complexity and disruptions in the field of regulated pharmaceutical products and medical devices, companies and regulatory authorities have been facing problems to find a skilled regulatory workforce (Drago et al., 2016). These undetected failures on regulatory systems lead to increased costs and poor productivity (Scannell et al., 2012).

Thus, the regulatory workforce must be capable of developing/applying strategies to protect the population from a hypothetical harmful medicinal product, as well as to ensure that favorable risk-benefit products are approved and available for all (Callréus & Schneider, 2013). The demand in the industry leads to the emergence of the concept of regulatory science. Although regulatory science still lacks an official definition, in the last decades a broader definition has appeared.

In 2007, The FDA defined "regulatory science" as *a science-based decision-making process needed to fulfill the responsibilities of a public health agency* ("Build. a Natl. Framew. Establ. Regul. Sci. Drug Dev.," 2011).

In 2009, Margaret Hamburg, FDA Commissioner affirmed that "regulatory science" is *the science and tools we use to assess and evaluate a product's safety* (Institute of Medicine (US) Forum on Drug Discovery Development and Translation, 2011).

The NIH-FDA collaboration to Fast-Track Innovations to the Public point of view on "regulatory science" is *The development and use of new tools, standards and approaches to more efficiently develop products and to more effectively evaluate product safety, efficacy and quality* ("Build. a Natl. Framew. Establ. Regul. Sci. Drug Dev.," 2011) (Food and Drug Administration, 2011).

EMA defined "regulatory science" as *the range of scientific disciplines that are applied to the quality, safety and efficacy assessment of medicinal products and that inform regulatory decision-making throughout the lifecycle of a medicine. It encompasses basic and applied biomedical and social sciences and contributes to the development of regulatory standards and tools* (European Medicines Agency, 2020a).

There are also other interesting definitions such as the one from Barry Coller. According to his point of view, "regulatory science" is a subset of the translational science, i.e. Coller affirms that "translational science" is *The application of the scientific method to address a health need and "regulatory science" is The application of the scientific method to improve the development, review, and oversight of new drugs, biologics, and devices that require regulatory approval before dissemination* ("Build. a Natl. Framew. Establ. Regul. Sci. Drug Dev.," 2011)

The president of the Institute for Regulatory Science, Alan Moghissi affirmed that *regulatory science is a unique application of science, at all levels, to the societal decision process* ("Build. a Natl. Framew. Establ. Regul. Sci. Drug Dev.," 2011).

Jeffrey Drazen, Editor-in-Chief of the New England Journal of Medicine and Co-Chair of the Drug Forum, described "regulatory science" as *a science that has been evolving and is continuing to evolve, but it's not as hard science as we would like* ("Build. a Natl. Framew. Establ. Regul. Sci. Drug Dev.," 2011).

Because biomedical and related sciences are in constant and fast development, a regulatory science program should be formed by a multidisciplinary program, including a dynamic broad of contents related to the acquisition of competencies in the fields of Biostatistics, decision theory, and information technology; Fundamentals of pharmacology; Scientific methodology; CT design; Drug, and device discovery and development; Clinical research; Monitoring, and quality assurance; Food, drug, and device law and regulation (Moghissi et al., 2020).

An exploratory study conducted by USA researchers to better understand the gaps and needs of pharmacy schools reported that students feeling a lack of acceptance of a "culture of safety", had difficulties in effectively communicate with patients and other healthcare providers about medication safety, a deficient knowledge on drug research and development process, as well as lack of skills to measure, build, or change a system to reduce errors and improve quality (Warholak et al., 2011). Moreover, according to the European students' perspective, European pharmacy lectures displayed some gaps that need to be improved, such as (a) students-professor communication, (b) lack of soft-skill sessions, (c) internships in industries, hospitals, pharmaceutical companies, laboratories, and insurance agencies, (d) lack of connection to a CT, regulatory affairs, and quality analysis, among others (European Pharmaceutical Students' Association, n.d.).

A recent study evaluated the existing program on regulatory science in the USA and observed that, although the educational programs complied with FDA regulations, some improvements are still needed, and for this reason, the authors suggested an outline for regulatory science education. (Moghissi et al., 2020).

Even though European universities have implemented the regulatory science program, according to our knowledge, no evaluation has been made to these programs. Recently, the Coordination and Support Action on Strengthening Training of Academia in Regulatory Science (CSA STARS) was implemented in 18 European countries, aiming to analyze and improve the training of academia in regulatory sciences, both at national and European levels (Strengthening Training of Academia in Regulatory Science (CSA STARS), n.d.).

Besides that, the European Pharmaceutical Students Organization (EPSA), involving all European pharmaceutical students' associations and represented by more than 100,000 students in 36 European countries, developed "the methodology booklet project", to collect pharmaceutical students and recent graduates' opinion on teaching methodologies around Europe and sharing these with educators (European Pharmaceutical Students' Association, n.d.).

REGULATORY SCIENCE AND REGULATORY AFFAIRS

According to experts, the development of an efficient regulatory workforce is essential to enhance the successful development of medical products and to ensure an improvement in the safety of the populations. Therefore, some academic institutions have already incorporated the field of regulatory science into their programs (Drago et al., 2016; Lumpkin et al., 2012; "Strength. a Work. Innov. Regul. Sci. Ther. Dev.," 2012; Tominaga et al., 2011).

In order to ensure protection and promote the health of the global population, in 2011, the FDA developed a regulatory science strategy based on seven keystones: (a) improving product safety through the modernization of toxicology (b) promoting clinical evaluation and personalized medicine modernization; (c) improving the quality and manufacturing of products; (d) guaranteeing a faster evaluation of new emerging technologies; (e) improving health outcomes through the analyses of the diverse scientific data; (f) creating a prevention-focused food safety system (g) promoting global health and security through the development of medical countermeasures; (h) promoting both consumers' and professionals' informed decisions through the strengthening of social and behavioral sciences. To achieve these goals, the FDA awarded four Centers of Excellence in Regulatory Science and Innovation (CERSIs) at academic institutions (Adamo et al., 2015; Hamburg, 2011).

In March 2020, EMA adopted the "Regulatory Science to 2025" strategy, based on the synergistic relationship between EMA, the European medicine regulatory network, and several academic research centers, with the following five main goals: (a) to promote the integration of science and technology in medicines development; (b) to improve the scientific quality of evaluations; (c) to encourage advancing patient-centered access to medicines in partnership with healthcare systems, (d) to address emerging health threats and availability/therapeutic challenges; (e) to promote the research and innovation in regulatory science (European Medicines Agency, 2020a; Food and Drug Administration, 2011; P. A. Hines et al., 2019).

New Approach to Learning Methodologies

There are different teaching-learning methodologies, disseminated by different countries/educational institutions, which have long been identified with a more traditional teaching methodology that emerged in Europe, in the 18th century. In this type of methodology, the transmission of information occurred hierarchically – from professor to student – with the students' progress being measured by periodic assessments.

The main goal was to provide the student with a solid base of information, leaving him to absorb the passively transmitted knowledge, memorizing it, especially through lectures, although there was no appreciation of how the students acquired their knowledge (Balardim, 2020; Dos et al., 2017). In the 60-70s, this methodology started to be seen as outdated. However, it continued to be adopted in numerous institutions all over the world, but increasingly combined with active learning methods.

In the last decades, several alternatives have been created to replace this traditional teaching method. Numerous articles have been published in the literature highlighting evidence that active learning produces better educational results than the traditional methodology based on lectures, as well as the recognition and appreciation of the construction and acquisition processes of knowledge by the students, thus allowing their involvement and active participation in this path (Dos et al., 2017; Kibble et al., 2016).

This active learning methodology constitutes a rupture with the teaching concepts most commonly found at the educational institutions. In this methodology, the student is the learning center, so he is not just listening and taking notes, he debates, criticizes, does, helps to build the knowledge together with the professor and his colleagues (Balardim, 2020).

Promoting and stimulating the development of learning skills throughout life, such as problem-solving and critical thinking, has become a crucial goal for higher education in the 21st century. According to the Bologna Declaration, successful learning and study in higher education must involve students in learning (Asikainen, 2014).

This active learning is becoming more common in undergraduate education in science, technology, engineering, and mathematics. According to a 2014 meta-analysis, there was an average increase of 6% in performance in evaluations, with students in courses based on traditional methods having about 1.5 times more probability to fail (Freeman et al., 2014). This active learning model is widely used in the health sciences field. However, it is important to note that the discussion around these teaching methods continues, there are no clear answers to more nuanced questions, such as: "How much active learning is enough?" or "What is the best type of active learning?" (Dos et al., 2017).

There are several models available, with the most common being problem-based learning (PBL), team-based learning (TBL) and, more recently, hybrid-PBL (h-PBL). The h-PBL model incorporates elements of both traditional methods and PBL for an increased teaching and education promotion in biomedical sciences (Jiménez-Saiz & Rosace, 2019).

The PBL method was introduced in the late 1960s, at the McMaster University in Canada, in the medicine course (Savery, 2006). In the 1970s, one of the European universities with the greatest visibility in this area, the University of Maastricht (UM), adopted the use of PBL aiming to integrate theoretical and practical knowledge, improve motivation and promote reasoning skills and more guided and independent learning (Jansen, 2019).

This learning model has, as its key element, problem-based learning, especially in small groups of students, since there is no single PBL. It is expected that the student is able to develop his personal, social and professional skills, with the university having the major role of preparing the student to live, work and contribute to society, through the development of his academic skills.

In this methodology, students acquire knowledge by discussing professionally relevant problems, therefore improving their application and integration. This method is supposed to encourage them to a deep learning approach, in which students try to understand and are intrinsically interested in what is being studied.

Another methodology, namely TBL, is a teaching method targeted to small groups, where students are guided to apply conceptual knowledge through a recurring sequence of activities that involve individual work, teamwork, and immediate feedback (Kibble et al., 2016). Unlike other methods targeted at small groups, a single expert on the subject can simultaneously be a facilitator of small groups of students working in a large classroom. TBL was created in the 1970s and is currently a well-documented and accepted teaching method, validated through its adoption by many disciplines in many countries worldwide (Haidet et al., 2012). Health professions are among those who have adopted this methodology the most, mostly due to their high concern in training professionals who are able to think critically and efficiently apply the concepts acquired in practice.

Regarding the h-PBL concept, understood as a combination of PBL and traditional methods, it is not an unforeseen situation. In fact, h-PBL has been used in a series of biomedical programs that are in transition from traditional to PBL, in courses where the traditional method is deeply rooted and the faculty professors do not support a pure PBL system, as well as by researchers genuinely interested in investigating h-PBL learning outcomes (Jiménez-Saiz & Rosace, 2019). Interestingly, many of the students reported their wish to attend lectures, at least sometimes, which indicates the need for more guidance. Thus, PBL tutors highlight the need to adapt PBL to the student's knowledge and complement it with guided sessions (for example, lectures). This suggests that guided lecture-based sessions could be a useful teaching tool to fill certain gaps in the PBL curriculum (Haghparast et al., 2007; Herdeiro et al., 2014).

Self-directed learning (SDL), also called self-education, andragogy, self-planned study, lifelong study, or autodidacticism, is a teaching autonomous methodology frequently found in universities worldwide. (Almeman & Alrebish, 2018). In this methodology, professors help the students to find a topic and study objectives, and then the students are free to build their own curriculum. The basic principle of this methodology is offering the student the opportunity to acquire sophisticated abilities and to become an evaluator of his knowledge (Kasworm, 2011). This methodology is influenced by the behaviors and cultural environment of the students.

New Methodologies in Pharmaceutical Sciences Curriculum

The use of teaching-learning methodologies is important within pharmaceutical sciences education, with several of these methods being applied in this teaching area. An article published in 2014 (Sugihara, 2014) refers to the adoption of learning strategies that were considered appropriate in classes, such as small discussion groups, World Café, and TBL and PBL tutorials. This study found that, although students were attracted by these methods, the difficulty in evaluation caused by the ambiguity on criteria may jeopardize the teaching program.

Another article published in 2019, aiming to redesign the pharmacology discipline, showed an increased active-learning when a portion of the time previously devoted to lecturing was replaced with an active-learning session.

This experience can serve as a blueprint for how to convert a lecture-only course into a hybrid lecture and recitation model (Hirvonen et al., 2019; Kennedy, 2019; Nachtigal et al., 2017; Petkova & Atkinson, 2017; Volmer et al., 2019). Another review published in 2015 addressed how the shift in the pharmacists' role, from simply dispensing medications to the effective delivery of pharmaceutical care interventions and drug therapy management, has influenced pharmacy education.

The educational focus has shifted from basic sciences to clinical and integrated courses that require incorporating active-learning strategies (as, for example, educational games) to provide pharmacy graduates with higher levels of competencies and specialized skills (Aburahma & Mohamed, 2015).

This teaching-learning model, which integrates an active methodology and/or a traditional and active methodology, is described as being good in the Health Sciences field, areas in which it is essential to integrate theoretical and practical knowledge and solve problems. These learning methods are mentioned in the fields of pharmacology, therapeutics, drug development, and the development of soft skills in the management of drug therapy (Aburahma & Mohamed, 2015).

Regulatory Affairs Pharmacists

Due to the growing need for highly qualified professionals in the field of regulatory affairs, one of the expertise areas of the pharmaceutical activity, which is highly competitive and challenging due to constant changes in the regulatory level, the Order of Pharmacists created the college of specialty in regulatory affairs, aiming to respond to the requirements of the global market, as well as to contribute for a high demand and quality standards of these professionals. This title of specialist has been awarded since 1998 and has so far 144 specialists (2019) (*Diário Da República - Normas Para Atribuição Do Título de Especialista Em Assuntos Regulamentares*, 2018).

Given the growing demand from regulatory authorities regarding the development and commercialization of health products, namely drugs for both human and veterinary use, medical devices, cosmetics, and other health products, both pre- and post-marketing, the regulatory affairs pharmacist assumes a predominant role in the pharmaceutical industry. To exercise the profession in regulatory affairs, pharmacists must have an in-depth knowledge of the legislation in force, allowing them to issue opinions based on technical and legal issues related to: (*APREFAR - APREFAR - Associação Dos Profissionais de Registos e Regulamentação Farmacêutica*, n.d.)

- Obtaining a MA, monitoring, and maintenance.
- Drug prices and reimbursement.
- Drug and medical devices' promotion, distribution, and sale.

This knowledge is essential to intervene from the earliest phase of chemical and pharmaceutical development of new products until pre-clinical and clinical research phases so that all legislative and ethical procedures are fulfilled, allowing the construction of the Common Technical Document to be submitted to the authorities.

The activities to be performed by the Regulatory Affairs professional in the Post-MA are also crucial, namely in terms of requesting for price and reimbursement, in participating in the maintenance procedures of MA, as well as in the post-marketing surveillance to ensure drug effectiveness and safety.

Thus, the Order of Pharmacists advocates as core competencies of the Specialist Pharmacist in Regulatory Affairs, the framing of activities in the following areas:

- Pharmaceutical regulatory context.
- Health systems.
- Pharmaceutical and health market.
- Good regulatory practices.
- Pharmaceutical research.
- Leadership and ethics.

*Regulatory knowledge and the development of activities underlying each functional area are essential for the development of competencies in these areas (*Diário Da República - Normas Para Atribuição Do Título de Especialista Em Assuntos Regulamentares, *2018)*

During the Integrated Master in Pharmaceutical Sciences (MICF) course, the pharmacist develops transversal skills in the fields of pharmaceutical development and preclinical and clinical research.

Table 1. Functional areas on regulatory affairs

Functional Area	Contents
Pharmaceutical Regulatory Context	• Regulatory agencies. • Regulatory context of other health products (medical devices, homeopathic products, dietary supplements, dietetics, and biocides). • Registration strategy; Forms and Pharmacopoeias. • National and European System of Pharmacovigilance. • Post-marketing surveillance and risk management. • European regulatory system and others. • Legislative texts.
Health Systems	• Pharmacoeconomics and Health Economics Studies. • Organization and financing of the NHS and other health systems. • Prices, co-payments.
Pharmaceutical and Health Market	• Market access and pre-launch actions. • Industrial, patients and other associations. • Hospital calls for tenders. • Drug distribution. • Business organization. • Organization, value and market segmentation. • Patents and registered trademarks. • Promotion and advertising of drugs and other health products. • Customer services (i.e. providing regulatory information to external and internal customers).
Good Regulatory Practices	• Pharmaceutical Regulation Activity. • MA for medicines and introduction health products on the market. • Archive, information systems. • Drug and health products' life cycle. • Compliance and notification of drug and health products' promotion. • Export/Import. • Authorizations for special and exceptional use. • Pharmacovigilance and post-marketing surveillance. • Crisis management and support with regulatory impact. • Regulatory quality, audit, quality systems. • Summary of product characteristics, Information leaflets, and labeling of drugs and health products.• Preparation and/or monitoring of the process of co-payment and economic evaluation. • Electronic submission.
Research and Development (medicines and health products)	• Clinical Trials. • Interpretation of scientific articles. • Galenic, pre-clinical and clinical research and development. • Drug quality. • Drugs' safety and efficacy.
Leadership and ethics	• Training activities. • Deontological codes. • Communication management. • Crisis management. • Departmental management. • Human resources leadership. • Pharmaceutical liability.

Source: Adapted from Diário Da República - Normas Para Atribuição Do Título de Especialista Em Assuntos Regulamentares, 2018

In Portugal, there are several public (N=5) and private (N=4) faculties/schools institutions offering the MICF. Besides these institutions, there are also preparatory courses in Pharmaceutical Sciences at the University of the Azores (*Acesso Ao Ensino Superior 2020 - Índices de Cursos (Por Curso e Instituição)*, n.d.). The MICF complies with the European Directive 2013/55/CE, enabling the Master to carry out all the activities included in the Pharmaceutical Act, being recognized by the Order of Pharmacists. All MICF study plans have a duration of 5 years and 300 ECTS (European Commission, 2013).

Regarding the curricular units (CU) in the field of regulatory affairs and clinical research, there has been an introduction of these CUs in the MICF curriculum in recent years, especially in the last two academic years (4th and 5th years), both as mandatory or optional subject.

At the European level, there are several courses on regulatory affairs, namely Masters' Degrees and expert courses, focuses on aspects regarding registration of medicines, as well as on all the technical requirements for the MA of the products (CESIF, 2020). The Universities of Copenhagen, Basel, Hertfordshire, Kings' College and others, have also collaborated in harmonizing programs to produce a common Masters' degree program in Medicines Regulatory Affairs, to be part of the PharmaTrain, an IMI Education & Training project (Medical University of Vienna, n.d.; ScanBalt, 2013; University of Copenhagen, 2020).

At the national level, the offer is also highly diversified in the various Portuguese universities, at the masters level, for instance, the master in "Regulation and Evaluation of Medicines and Health Products" from the Faculty of Pharmacy of the University of Lisbon, or in "Clinical Research Management" from both the Nova University of Lisbon and the University of Aveiro; as well as at the postgraduate level, for example, postgraduate courses in "Pharmaceutical and Parapharmaceutical Industry", in "Clinical Trials and Medical Affairs Monitoring", an open specialization program in "Project Management in Clinical Research", among other specialization courses held by several Contract Research Organization (CRO), and also by some universities.

Clinical Studies Research

Clinical research, in particular CTs, is also an area of intervention and an opportunity for pharmacists with competencies in the regulatory field to be able to exercise their activity.

A document published by the Portuguese Pharmaceutical Industry Association (APIFARMA) in 2019 states that the development of CTs has an unquestionable significant impact on the social and economic levels in the country where they are performed (APIFARMA, 2019; European Commission, 2020). In addition to the economic impact, the development of this activity also contributes to the deepening of fundamental knowledge for healthcare improvement, thus facilitating early access to innovative medicines and the increase of professionals in the sector, among others.

CTs should be designed, conducted, and analyzed in concordance with scientific principles, and should be reported appropriately. Essentially, the rationale of drug development is to ask important questions and subsequently to answer them with appropriate studies. Classically, clinical drug development is often described as consisting of four temporal phases (Phase I-IV), presented in Figure 1 (International conference on harmonization of technical requirements for registration of pharmaceuticals for human use, 1997).

Figure 1. Schematic representation of the clinical trials' phases
Source: Food and Drug Administration, 2018 - https://www.fda.gov/patients/drug-development-process/step-3-clinical-research)

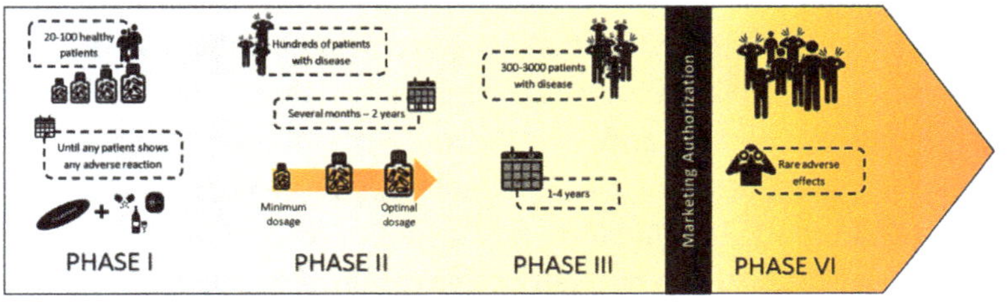

At the European level and according to the European Commission (EC) in 2018, the pharmaceutical industry was the sector with the largest volume of investment in R&D worldwide (€ 153.8 billion), and the greatest intensity of R&D, as the weight of the R&D value on industry sales/business is 15.4% (APIFARMA, 2019; European Commission, 2020).

The main stakeholders involved in CTs are patients, sponsors, regulatory authorities (ethics and competent authorities), hospital administration boards, CT sites of recruitment, research teams, and CRO. In Portugal, the performance of CTs is subject to strict regulation. The new European Regulation No. 536/2014 (RE), on CTs for medicines for human use, which will come into force in the coming years, introduces the procedures to be followed by all member states, as well as the national competencies of each state member. The RE will coexist with the national legislation of each country (European Commission, 2020).

To conduct a CT, it is necessary not only the intervention of those responsible for the study (applicants, sponsors, and researchers) and the subjects' written consent but also the accomplishment of a series of lengthy requirements and procedures for the study to be validated and later started, in order to apply GCP concepts. After the design of the study is finished, the applicant must submit the request for the CT to INFARMED and the Ethics Committee for Clinical Research (CEIC, 2016).

Within the scope of the SIMPLEX+ Program, on December 5th, 2016, the National Registry of Clinical Studies (RNEC) emerged, with the main objective of simplifying, modernizing, and streamlining processes and promoting transparency, following the Resolution of the Council of Ministers no. 56/2016, published in Diário da República on October 13th, which approved the National Strategy for Medicines and Health Products 2016-2020 (SNS, 2017).

The lack of CT registration platforms, such as EudraCT in Europe and Clinicaltrials.gov in the United States, was associated with several problems, mainly in terms of selectivity in reporting CTs.

Currently, the ClinicalTrials.gov registration platform, created in 2000, has more than 325,000 registered CTs, and the EudraCT platform, established in 2004, has more than 36,000 registered trials.

The RNEC consists of a public register of CTs that are in the most diverse stages and is a support for conducting CTs (INFARMED, 2016). This platform (SNS, 2016) is intended for the following trials:

- CTs with medicinal products for human use;
- Clinical studies involving medical devices;
- Clinical studies involving cosmetic products;
- Post-Authorization Effectiveness Studies (PAES) without intervention;
- Post-Authorization Security Studies (PASS) without intervention.

This platform has a public area, accessible to all citizens, where all information related to CTs in Portugal is available throughout its various stages, namely the identification of trial centers, sponsors, and other information related to the trial. Moreover, the possibility to search for entities and individuals associated with clinical research, such as sponsors, researchers, monitors, etc, is also available (SNS, 2016).

The Clinical Research Law (*Lei n.º 21/2014, de 16 de Abril*, 2014) defines disclosure of a clinical study as *any form of communication that has the purpose or effect of reporting on the conduction of a clinical study, which may include observations made in the context of the study, interpretation of results and conclusions of the same with the public, with health professionals, with the media, in general, or scientific publications, regardless of its target audience, and in advertising material for medicines, medical devices or any other means of intervention in health*, and states that the dissemination of clinical studies can be done by the researcher, the research team or intermediaries.

The dissemination of clinical studies to the public must be identified as such, expressly indicating that it is a clinical study and has to be approved by CEIC previously to the disclosure. (*Lei n.º 21/2014, de 16 de Abril*, 2014; SNS, 2016).

The graph below, presented in Figure 2, taken from the document "Statistics for the evaluation of clinical trials by INFARMED", clearly shows the discrepancy in the percentages between the phases I/II and phase III trials (INFARMED, 2017).

Figure 2. Clinical trials statistics
Source: INFARMED, 2017

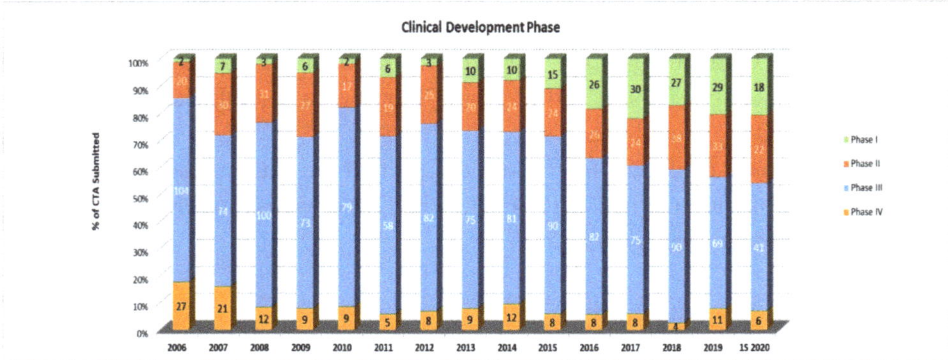

Figure 3. Clinical trial applications
Source: INFARMED, 2017

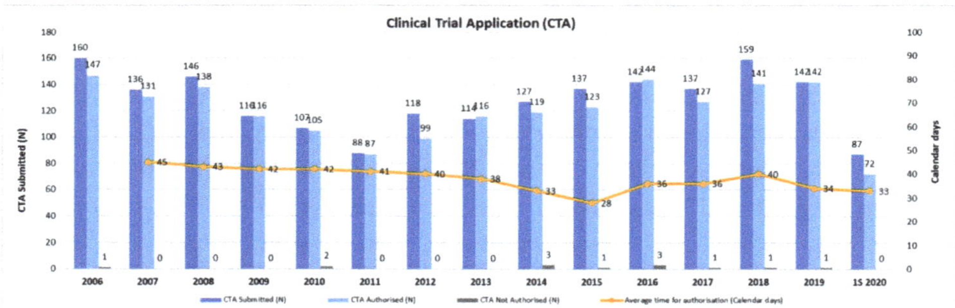

According to INFARMED data regarding CTs only (Figure 3) have remained constant since 2016, with a slight increase in 2018, but not yet reaching the value of 2006 (n = 160 PAEC). Concerning clinical development phases, it is phase III that presents a greater number of requests, despite having been decreasing. On the other hand, phases I and II have been increasing slightly (INFARMED, 2017).

Risk Management, Pharmacovigilance and European Project Networks

Pharmacovigilance, one of the main activities presented throughout the medicines' life cycle is defined by WHO (2002) as *the science and activities relating to the detection, assessment, understanding, and prevention of adverse drug effects or any other possible drug-related problem.* From the regulatory point of view, it is *the activity developed with the goal of enabling the identification and investigation of safety problems related to medicines, in a fast and effective way, together with the implementation of suitable measures for the protection of Public Health.*

The safety of medicines is one of the fundamental principles in its evaluation, either in pre-MA and post-MA, being thus included in the contents of several of the functional fields for awarding the title of specialist in regulatory affairs (see Table 1).

Several projects have been launched to improve both the science and practice of pharmacovigilance. One example is the joint action Strengthening Collaboration for Operating Pharmacovigilance in Europe (SCOPE), strengthening the collaboration of pharmacovigilance in Europe, the European Network of Centers for Pharmacoepidemiology and Pharmacovigilance (ENCePP), that incorporates centers for pharmacoepidemiology and pharmacovigilance, and Pharmacoepidemiological Research on Outcomes of Therapeutics by a European Consortium (PROTECT) (Pêgo et al., 2018).

In general, the practice of pharmacovigilance and regulatory affairs demands highly qualified professionals and extremely organized institutions.

SOLUTIONS AND RECOMMENDATIONS

The faculties/schools of pharmacy must be able to anticipate or rapidly adapted its teaching methodologies according to the demands of the market and the needs of the population.

In this context, new teaching methodologies should be introduced within the curriculum to implement new competencies, such as communication skills, teamwork, self-learning, etc. A compromise among traditional and new strategies of learning such as PBL, SDL and TBL should be found to guarantee the acquisition of skills for a successful pharmacist's profession.

Nevertheless, pharmacy faculties/schools must keep in mind that the initial education of pharmacists should still cover the fundamental sciences that give them the proper knowledge and competencies to be involved in technical and scientific work. Clinical research and regulatory science are a very crucial phase of education when pharmacists can use their skills efficiently. Therefore, to become an expert in a specific field, postgraduate courses should be provided in collaboration with experts working in pharmaceutical institutions, aiming to help students be more proficient.

A close relationship among the pharmaceutical industry, CRO, government agencies, and pharmacy faculties/schools should be promoted, by instance through internships, to facilitate the acquisition of skills related to a CT, drug development, and regulatory science.

FUTURE RESEARCH DIRECTIONS

There are countless theories regarding the best strategy to learn. Nevertheless, it is imperative to take in mind that optimal learning or teaching style is dependent on the students' needs and the environment.

Since the pharmaceutical industry/CRO/regulatory authorities are increasing the demand for more specialized and differentiated pharmacists, we believed that new methodologies focused on developing individual skills and increasing the motivation of pharmacists will be crucial to enhance the success of pharmacists and ensure an efficient and robust workforce.

CONCLUSION

We found that promotion and development of dynamic learning have been embraced in pharmacy faculties/schools, based on both students' preferences and market demands. In this context, worldwide strategies have been adopted to guarantee that students efficiently develop skills in regulatory affairs and clinical research.

However, some efforts still need to be employed to ensure a more coherent pharmacist education among European countries, to enable students' mobility and also to improve pharmacist skills across Europe.

ACKNOWLEDGMENT

We thank Ana Plácido, PhD., Tânia Magalhães Silva, PhD., and Marta Estrela, MSc., for their collaboration on this chapter.

This research was supported by the APIMedOlder project [PTDC/MED-FAR/31598/2017] and by the eHealthResp project [PTDC/SAU-SER/31678/2017], funded by the operational program of competitiveness and internationalization (POCI), in its FEDER/FNR component POCI-01-0145-FEDER-031598 and POCI-01-0145-FEDER-031678, respectively, and the Foundation for Science and Technology (Fundação Para a Ciência e Tecnologia - FCT), in its state budget component (OE).

REFERENCES

Aburahma, M. H., & Mohamed, H. M. (2015). Educational games as a teaching tool in pharmacy curriculum. American Journal of Pharmaceutical Education. doi:10.5688/ajpe79459

Acesso ao Ensino Superior 2020 - Índices de Cursos (por curso e instituição). (n.d.). Retrieved September 30, 2020, from https://www.dges.gov.pt/guias/indcurso.asp?curso=9494

Adamo, J. E., Wilhelm, E. E., & Steele, S. J. (2015). Advancing a Vision for Regulatory Science Training. *Clinical and Translational Science*, *8*(5), 615–618. Advance online publication. doi:10.1111/cts.12298 PMID:26083660

Almeman, A. A., & Alrebish, S. A. (2018). Teaching Strategies Used in Pharmacy. In *Pharmacy Education in the Twenty First Century and Beyond* (pp. 125–145). Elsevier., doi:10.1016/B978-0-12-811909-9.00010-1

Altman, R. B., Khuri, N., Salit, M., & Giacomini, K. M. (2015). Unmet needs: Research helps regulators do their jobs. Science Translational Medicine. doi:10.1126citranslmed.aac4369

APIFARMA. (2019). *Ensaios clínicos em Portugal*. www.pwc.pt/s&cfa

APREFAR - APREFAR - Associação dos Profissionais de Registos e Regulamentação Farmacêutica. (n.d.). Retrieved October 1, 2020, from https://www.aprefar.pt/conteudos/?page=aprefar

Asikainen, H. (2014). *Successful learning and studying in biosciences*. University of Helsinky.

Balardim, G. (2020). *Metodologias de ensino: confira 10 das mais usadas nas escolas*. https://www.clipescola.com/metodologias-de-ensino-confira/

Brown, A. N., Gilbert, B. J., Bruno, A. F., & Cooper, G. M. (2012). Validated competency framework for delivery of pharmacy services in pacific-Island countries. *Journal of Pharmacy Practice and Research*. doi:10.1002/j.2055-2335.2012.tb00186.x

Building a National Framework for the Establishment of Regulatory Science for Drug Development. (2011). In *Building a National Framework for the Establishment of Regulatory Science for Drug Development*. doi:10.17226/12968

Callréus, T., & Schneider, C. K. (2013). The emergence of regulatory science in pharmaceutical medicine. Pharmaceutical Medicine. doi:10.100740290-013-0039-x

CEIC. (2016). *Ensaios Clínicos - Fluxograma de processo*. https://www.rnec.pt/submissao-nacional

CESIF. (2020). *Professional Expert Course Records and Regulatory Affairs*. https://www.healthcarestudies.com/Course-Professional-Expert-Drug-Registration-And-Regulatory-Affairs/Spain/CESIF/

Diário da República - Normas para atribuição do título de especialista em assuntos regulamentares. (2018) (testimony of Assembleia da República).

Dos, L., Lima, S., & Cosme, A. (2017). *A metodologia de ensino-aprendizagem-avaliação através da resolução de problemas: O recorte de uma tese em desenvolvimento*. https://repositorio-aberto.up.pt/bitstream/10216/119397/2/322923.pdf

Drago, D., Shire, S., & Ekmekci, O. (2016). Improving Regulatory Education: Can We Reconcile Employers' Expectations With Academic Offerings? *Therapeutic Innovation & Regulatory Science*, *50*(3), 330–336. Advance online publication. doi:10.1177/2168479015620440 PMID:30227069

Dreyfus, S. E. (2004). The five-stage model of adult skill acquisition. *Bulletin of Science, Technology & Society*, *24*(3), 177–181. Advance online publication. doi:10.1177/0270467604264992

European Commission. (2013). *Diretiva 2013/55/UE do Parlamento Europeu e do Conselho, de 20 de novembro de 2013, que altera a Diretiva 2005/36/CE relativa ao reconhecimento das qualificações profissionais e o Regulamento (UE) n.o 1024/2012 relativo à cooperação administrativa através*. Jornal Oficial Da União Europeia.

European Commission. (2020). *EU R&D Scoreboard*. doi:10.2760/59430

European Medicines Agency. (2020a). *Advancing regulatory science in the EU – new strategy adopted*. Author.

European Medicines Agency. (2020b). *Human regulatory*. Clinical Trial Regulation.

European Medicines Agency. (n.d.). *Clinical Trials*. Author.

European Pharmaceutical Students' Association. (n.d.). *Methodology Booklet*. Author.

Food and Drug Administration. (2011). *Moving Regulatory Science into the 21st Century*. Advancing Regulatory Science at FDA.

Food and Drug Administration. (2018). *Step 3: Clinical Research | FDA*. https://www.fda.gov/patients/drug-development-process/step-3-clinical-research

Food and Drug Administration. (2020). *FDA Regulations Relating to Good Clinical Practice and Clinical Trials. Regulations: Good Clinical Practice and Clinical Trials*. Author.

Frank, J. R., Mungroo, R., Ahmad, Y., Wang, M., De Rossi, S., & Horsley, T. (2010). Toward a definition of competency-based education in medicine: A systematic review of published definitions. *Medical Teacher*, *32*(8), 631–637. Advance online publication. doi:10.3109/0142159X.2010.500898 PMID:20662573

Freeman, S., Eddy, S. L., McDonough, M., Smith, M. K., Okoroafor, N., Jordt, H., & Wenderoth, M. P. (2014). Active learning increases student performance in science, engineering, and mathematics. *Proceedings of the National Academy of Sciences of the United States of America*. 10.1073/pnas.1319030111

Haghparast, N., Sedghizadeh, P. P., Shuler, C. F., Ferati, D., & Christersson, C. (2007). Evaluation of student and faculty perceptions of the PBL curriculum at two dental schools from a student perspective: A cross-sectional survey. *European Journal of Dental Education*, *11*(1), 14–22. Advance online publication. doi:10.1111/j.1600-0579.2007.00423.x PMID:17227391

Haidet, P., Levine, R. E., Parmelee, D. X., Crow, S., Kennedy, F., Kelly, P. A., Perkowski, L., Michaelsen, L., & Richards, B. F. (2012). Perspective: Guidelines for reporting team-based learning activities in the medical and health sciences education literature. Academic Medicine. doi:10.1097/ACM.0b013e318244759e

Hamburg, M. A. (2011). Advancing Regulatory Science. Science. doi:10.1126cience.1204432

Herdeiro, M. T., Teixeira Rodrigues, A., Ferreira, M., da Cruz e Silva, O. A. B., & Fardilha, M. (2014). Multi-method active learning approach: Improving the educational experience in pharmaceutical drug development. *Indian Journal of Pharmaceutical Education and Research*. doi:10.5530/ijper.48.3.4

Hines, P. A., Guy, R. H., Humphreys, A. J., & Papaluca-Amati, M. (2019). The European Medicines Agency's goals for regulatory science to 2025. Nature Reviews Drug Discovery. doi:10.1038/d41573-019-00071-2

Hines, P. A., Gonzalez-Quevedo, R., Lambert, A. I. O. M., Janssens, R., Freischem, B., Torren Edo, J., Claassen, I. J. T. M., & Humphreys, A. J. (2020). Regulatory Science to 2025: An Analysis of Stakeholder Responses to the European Medicines Agency's Strategy. *Frontiers in Medicine*, *7*, 508. Advance online publication. doi:10.3389/fmed.2020.00508 PMID:33072771

Hines, P. A., Guy, R. H., Brand, A., Humphreys, A. J., & Papaluca-Amati, M. (2019). Regulatory Science and Innovation Programme for Europe (ReScIPE): A proposed model. *Journal of Clinical Pharmacology*. PMID:31426120

Hirvonen, J., Salminen, O., Vuorensola, K., Katajavuori, N., Huhtala, H., & Atkinson, J. (2019). Pharmacy Practice and Education in Finland. *Pharmacy (Basel, Switzerland)*, *7*(1), 21. Advance online publication. doi:10.3390/pharmacy7010021 PMID:30813453

INFARMED. (2017). *Estatísticas de avaliação de ensaios clínicos pelo Infarmed.* https://www.infarmed.pt/web/infarmed/entidades/medicamentos-uso-humano/ensaios-clinicos/estatisticas

Institute of Medicine (US) Forum on Drug Discovery Development and Translation. (2011). *Building a National Framework for the Establishment of Regulatory Science for Drug Development: Workshop Summary*. Author.

International Conference on Harmonisation of Technical Requirements for Registration of Pharmaceuticals for Human Use. (1997). *General Considerations for Clinical Trials E8.* Author.

Ioannidis, J. P. A. (2016). Why Most Clinical Research Is Not Useful. *PLoS Medicine*, *13*(6), e1002049. Advance online publication. doi:10.1371/journal.pmed.1002049 PMID:27328301

Jansen, W. (2019). *Problem-based Learning at Maastricht University. Academic Press.*

Jiménez-Saiz, R., & Rosace, D. (2019). Is hybrid-PBL advancing teaching in biomedicine? A systematic review. BMC Medical Education. doi:10.118612909-019-1673-0

Kasworm, C. (2011). New perspectives on post-formal cognitive development and self-directed learning. *International Journal of Self-Directed Learning*, *8*(1).

Katoue, M. G., & Schwinghammer, T. L. (2020). Competency-based education in pharmacy: A review of its development, applications, and challenges. *Journal of Evaluation in Clinical Practice*, *26*(4), 1–10. doi:10.1111/jep.13362 PMID:32069376

Kennedy, D. R. (2019). Redesigning a pharmacology course to promote active learning. *American Journal of Pharmaceutical Education, 83*(5), 6782. Advance online publication. doi:10.5688/ajpe6782 PMID:31333258

Kibble, J. D., Bellew, C., Asmar, A., & Barkley, L. (2016). Team-based learning in large enrollment classes. *Advances in Physiology Education, 40*(4), 435–442. doi:10.1152/advan.00095.2016 PMID:27697956

Koster, A., Schalekamp, T., & Meijerman, I. (2017). Implementation of competency based pharmacy education (CBPE). *Pharmacy (Basel, Switzerland), 5*(1), 10. doi:10.3390/pharmacy5010010 PMID:28970422

Lei n.º 21/2014, de 16 de abril, (2014) (testimony of INFARMED). https://www.infarmed.pt/documents/15786/1068535/036-B1_Lei_21_2014_1alt.pdf

Lumpkin, M. M., Eichler, H. G., Breckenridge, A., Hamburg, M. A., Lönngren, T., & Woods, K. (2012). Advancing the science of medicines regulation: The role of the 21st-century medicines regulator. Clinical Pharmacology and Therapeutics. doi:10.1038/clpt.2012.146

Medical University of Vienna. (n.d.). *The MRA: European Master of Regulatory Affairs*. Retrieved October 1, 2020, from http://www.emtrain.eu/index.php/news/410-the-mra-european-master-of-regulatory-affairs

Moghissi, A., Calderone, R., Auffret, J. P., Jaeger, L., Longstreth, J., McBride, D., Steen, T., Harrison, D., Garrison, D., & McDaniel, N. (2020). Regulatory Science Education: The Need for Generalization. *Journal of Regional Science, 8*, 1–7.

Nachtigal, P., Šimůnek, T., & Atkinson, J. (2017). Pharmacy Practice and Education in the Czech Republic. *Pharmacy (Basel, Switzerland), 5*(4), 54. Advance online publication. doi:10.3390/pharmacy5040054 PMID:28991203

Pêgo, A., Pereira, A. da C., Figueiredo, A., Araújo, A., Severiano, A. I., Macedo, A., Anes, A. M., Silva, A. M., Moreira, A., Paróla, A., Duarte, A. P., Martins, A. P., Martins, A. S., Vaz, A. F., Lourenço, A., Gouveia, A. M., de Araújo, A. V. R., Torre, C., Ribeiro, C. F., . . . Maria, V. A. (2018). Farmacovigilância em Portugal: 25 anos. In *Farmacovigilância em Portugal: 25 anos*. http://app10.infarmed.pt/e_book_farmacovigilancia25/index.html

Petkova, V., & Atkinson, J. (2017). Pharmacy Practice and Education in Bulgaria. *Pharmacy (Basel, Switzerland), 5*(4), 35. Advance online publication. doi:10.3390/pharmacy5030035 PMID:28970446

Rasi, G. (2017). *EU's innovative medical technology and EMA's measures*. Symposium, Presented at Summit of Heads of Medicines Regulatory Agencies (ICMRA)., and International Coalition of Medicines Regulatory Authorities.

Savery, J. R. (2006). Overview of Problem-based Learning: Definitions and Distinctions. *The Interdisciplinary Journal of Problem-Based Learning, 1*(1). Advance online publication. doi:10.7771/1541-5015.1002

ScanBalt. (2013). *Four universities collaborate to introduce a European Masters Programme in Medicines Regulatory Affairs - Scanbalt*. https://scanbalt.org/scanbalt-news/four-universities-collaborate-introduce-european-masters-programme-medicines-regulatory-affairs/

Scannell, J. W., Blanckley, A., Boldon, H., & Warrington, B. (2012). Diagnosing the decline in pharmaceutical R&D efficiency. Nature Reviews Drug Discovery. doi:10.1038/nrd3681

SNS. (2016). *Registo Nacional de Estudos Clínicos (RNEC)*. https://www.rnec.pt/

SNS. (2017). *Registo Nacional de Estudos Clínicos (RNEC) – SNS*. https://www.sns.gov.pt/reforma-faq/registo-nacional-de-estudos-clinicos-rnec-6/

Strengthening a Workforce for Innovative Regulatory Science in Therapeutics Development. (2012). In *Strengthening a Workforce for Innovative Regulatory Science in Therapeutics Development*. doi:10.17226/13283

Strengthening Training of Academia in Regulatory Science (CSA STARS). (n.d.). Academic Press.

Sugihara, T. (2014). Current and ideal stages of pharmaceutical education. Yakugaku Zasshi. doi:10.1248/yakushi.14-00215-2

Tominaga, T., Asahina, Y., Uyama, Y., & Kondo, T. (2011). Regulatory science as a bridge between science and society. *Clinical Pharmacology and Therapeutics, 90*(1), 1–3. doi:10.1038/clpt.2011.89 PMID:21691273

University of Copenhagen. (2020). *European University Collaboration – University of Copenhagen*. https://mra.ku.dk/behind/pharmatrain/

Volmer, D., Sepp, K., Raal, A., & Atkinson, J. (2019). Pharmacy Practice and Education in Estonia. *Pharmacy (Basel, Switzerland), 7*(3), 87. Advance online publication. doi:10.3390/pharmacy7030087 PMID:31295797

Warholak, T. L., Holdford, D. A., West, D., Debake, D. L., Bentley, J. P., Malone, D. C., & Murphy, J. E. (2011). Perspectives on educating pharmacy students about the science of safety. *American Journal of Pharmaceutical Education*, *75*(7), 142. Advance online publication. doi:10.5688/ajpe757142 PMID:21969728

ADDITIONAL READING

Adamo, J. E., Wilhelm, E. E., & Steele, S. J. (2015). Advancing a Vision for Regulatory Science Training. *Clinical and Translational Science*, *8*(5), 615–618. Advance online publication. doi:10.1111/cts.12298 PMID:26083660

Almeman, A. A., & Alrebish, S. A. (2018). Teaching Strategies Used in Pharmacy. Pharmacy Education in the Twenty First Century and Beyond, 125–145. doi:10.1016/B978-0-12-811909-9.00010-1

European Medicines Agency. (2020b). EMA Regulatory Science to 2025. EMA/110706/2020. https://www.ema.europa.eu/en/documents/regulatory-procedural-guideline/ema-regulatory-science-2025-strategic-reflection_en.pdf

European Medicines Agency. (2020c). *Human regulatory*. Clinical Trial Regulation.

European Pharmaceutical Students' Association. (n.d.). Methodology Booklet. 2018.

FDA. (2018). Step 3: Clinical Research I FDA. https://www.fda.gov/patients/drug-development-process/step-3-clinical-research

Food and Drug Admnistration. (2020). FDA Regulations Relating to Good Clinical Practice and Clinical Trials. Regulations: Good Clinical Practice and Clinical Trials.

Hines, P. A., Gonzalez-Quevedo, R., Lambert, A. I. O. M., Janssens, R., Freischem, B., Torren Edo, J., Claassen, I. J. T. M., & Humphreys, A. J. (2020). Regulatory Science to 2025: An Analysis of Stakeholder Responses to the European Medicines Agency's Strategy. *Frontiers in Medicine*, *7*, 508. Advance online publication. doi:10.3389/fmed.2020.00508 PMID:33072771

Kennedy, D. R. (2019). Redesigning a pharmacology course to promote active learning. *American Journal of Pharmaceutical Education*, *83*(5), 6782. Advance online publication. doi:10.5688/ajpe6782 PMID:31333258

Moghissi, A., Calderone, R., Auffret, J. P., Jaeger, L., Longstreth, J., McBride, D., Steen, T., Harrison, D., Garrison, D., & McDaniel, N. (2020). Regulatory Science Education: The Need for Generalization. *Journal of Regional Science*, *8*, 1–7.

KEY TERMS AND DEFINITIONS

Clinical Research: Umbrella term encompassing all the investigations related to prevention, diagnosis, treatment, disease prognosis or health improvement.

Competency-Based Education (CBE): A teaching methodology that allows students' progression, mainly based on their skills and own perceptions of the surrounding environment. This methodology can lead to improved outcomes since the students develop their skills according to a societal healthcare need.

Regulatory Affairs: A profession essentially developed to protect public health by controlling the safety and efficacy of medicinal products in several areas, such as pharmaceuticals, veterinary medicines, medical devices, pesticides, agrochemicals, cosmetics and complementary medicines. The regulatory affairs professional must know regulatory science.

Regulatory Science: The science comprising scientific knowledge from a range of disciplines, including basic and applied medicinal sciences and social sciences, that develop policy measures to guarantee the quality, safety and efficacy assessment of medicinal products and that inform regulatory decision-making throughout the life cycle of a medicine, aiming to ensure the safety and well-being of the populations.

Chapter 9
Relationships Between Academia and Professionals:
The Contribution of the Portuguese Education and Practice Platform

Filipa Alves da Costa
Portuguese Pharmaceutical Society, Lisbon, Portugal

Maria Margarida Caramona
Faculty of Pharmacy, University of Coimbra, Portugal

ABSTRACT

Professional practice is regulated by associations with regulatory powers, namely the Portuguese Pharmaceutical Society (PPS). Education is regulated by the Ministry of Education, responsible for ensuring access to quality of education for all citizens across all professional spectra. Aiming to contribute to an improved continuity between education and the career pathway, from early phases to eventual specialization, the PPS, who represents the interests of all registered pharmacists, developed a new structure entitled the Education and Practice Platform (EPP). This structure includes one representative from each institution providing education in pharmaceutical sciences and all Councils of Specialty Boards of Practice. This chapter provides an overview of pharmacy education in Portugal, present the authors' view of strengths and limitation of the current educational system, and details the development of the EPP, presenting achievements to date, future plans, and expectations on the EPP's contribution on aligning education with societal needs.

DOI: 10.4018/978-1-7998-4486-0.ch009

INTRODUCTION

Society has been changing its disease patterns, most markedly over the last century. In industrialized countries and progressing globally, non-communicable diseases play a growing role, leading to different care needs. Citizens and consumers are also becoming constantly more demanding, again impacting on care provision. All these factors call for responsive systems of education that can prepare pharmacists for the new demands of the profession.

This chapter will start by providing a historical perspective on pharmacy education in Portugal; presenting the current challenges that academia faces to answer societal requests and demands from the employers in the pharmaceutical sector. We will then describe the development of an initiative developed within the Pharmaceutical Society, which aims to contribute to better alignment between education and practice. We shall present our views on the way this platform may contribute in the present and possibly in the future to motivate stakeholders involved to find common interests and share possible joint solutions for more competent pharmacists to better meet the current societal needs.

The main objectives of this text are therefore to provide an overview of pharmacy education in Portugal, comment on the changes in the pharmaceutical workforce to meet societal needs; while highlighting some identified gaps in education and practice, and finally concluding on how a structure like the education and practice platform may contribute to further align workforce demands with the academic offer.

The specific objectives are to:

- Describe current pharmacy education globally and in Portugal.
- Highlight opportunities for improvements in education.
- Describe the current pharmaceutical workforce, demands, and needs globally and in Portugal.
- Highlight opportunities for improvement in practice.
- Define the common interests of academia and pharmacy professionals.
- Describe the developments within the Platform Education and Practice as a contribution to some of these factors.

BACKGROUND

Historical Perspective on Pharmacy Education in Portugal

Pharmacy education in Portugal dates to the XVI century, in the University of Coimbra. There were specific courses for the so-called "apothecaries". However, pharmaceutical sciences as a high-level degree were only formally recognized at the beginning of the XIX century. In the XX century, pharmacy graduates could study for three years in one of three Schools of Pharmacy, Oporto, Coimbra and Lisbon, to become bachelors and then, if wanting to become pharmacists and having an average grade over 14 out of 20, they would take another two years, only available in Oporto.

This situation persisted until the sixties, and only since then the three Schools became recognized as University Education. Before 1992, only these three publicly subsidized faculties existed but as the course became more popular and prominent, with many students annually being left out because of insufficient placements, private faculties started to emerge.

Currently, there are nine faculties of pharmacy in Portugal, five publicly funded and four private; distributed through the mainland from North to South of the country.

Regulation of Pharmacy Education

The Bologna Declaration signed in 1999 by the ministers responsible for higher education in 29 European countries, was an inter-governmental agreement to reform higher education at the European level. This agreement was inspired by the objectives of the Lisbon Strategy, leading to the creation of the European Higher Education Area (EHEA), which aims to be an open area where students and graduates can benefit from mobility and fair access, without obstacles, to high-level quality education.

The core bases are mutual recognition of diplomas and other higher education qualifications, transparency (readable and comparable degrees organized in a three-cycle structure) and European cooperation on quality assurance. The EHEA currently comprises 48 signatories, nearly all the European countries (European Higher Education Area, 2019).

This implies courses have a common structure and then enable the transfer of credit units to another degree or another country. Since then, the course of Pharmaceutical Sciences is named as an Integrated Master, which is an integrated study cycle combining first and second cycle levels and obeys to a European Credit Transfer and Accumulation System (ECTS). The ECTS is a student-centered system based on the student workload required to achieve the objectives of a program of study. These objectives should preferably be specified in terms of learning outcomes and competencies to be acquired. ECTS is based on the principle that 60 credits measure the workload of a full-time student during one academic year. The student workload of a full-time study program in Europe amounts in most cases to around 1500-1800 hours per year and in those cases, one credit stands for around 25 to 30 working hours. Sensibly, 30 credits correspond to a study semester and 20 credits to a study trimester (Law Decree 42/2005, de 22nd February).

The use of the ECTS is common to various areas of study leading students to practice specific professions, including pharmacists, dentists, medical doctors but also non-health-related occupations such as engineers. In this level of education, it is compulsory that in addition to the curricular units covered throughout the nine semesters (accumulating 300 ECTS), there is a practical internship and an internship report or an original thesis. This internship period for pharmacists is normally completed during 10 to 12 weeks in community or hospital pharmacy, according to the demands of the European directive, and grants the additional of 30-36 ECTS. In some faculties, both the report and the thesis are demanded. Upon successful completion of the full study cycle, the student becomes a Master in Pharmaceutical Sciences, becoming professionally qualified and ready to register in the Pharmaceutical Society.

Accreditation of Pharmacy Education

Traditionally, education was foreseen by the Ministry of Education, but since 2000, there was the institution of the European Network for Quality Assurance in Higher Education, renamed as European Association for Quality Assurance in Higher Education in 2004 (ENQA).

The ENQA aims to disseminate good higher educational practices and as such contribute to ensuring quality. The creation of such an agency led to the development of a new method for accrediting education in many countries, including Portugal.

Currently, the accreditation of a study cycle consists of the verification of the compliance of the requirements that are necessary for a study cycle to be created and fully operational. In Portugal, this procedure is carried out by the Agency for Assessment and Accreditation of Higher Education (A3ES).

The most recent cycle of an evaluation carried out by the A3ES was finalized in 2018 and consisted of a thorough and exhaustive assessment of the nine degrees and faculties existing in the country. During the assessment, various national and international experts are called to provide their views and opinions on the extent to which each degree meets the accreditation requirements.

The general requirements for the accreditation of a study cycle are:

1. An education, scientific and cultural project adequate to the aims of the study cycle.
2. Qualified teaching staff.
3. Human and material resources necessary to ensure the level and quality of the program, namely adequate education and research facilities, equipment, libraries and laboratories.

In the pharmaceutical arena, this implies that the project reflects the adequate level for integrated masters, through which there is evidence of in-depth knowledge acquisition (e.g. understanding of pathophysiology), but also evidence of research development (e.g. development of new compounds or pharmaceutical formula) and fostering of critical thinking competencies (e.g. case-solving).

In practice, it means that the degree should reflect a good balance of structural units but also advanced practice units where translational knowledge is possible. It also implies a good ratio of pharmacist versus non-pharmacists teaching staff and that the educational degree of the teaching staff is appropriate to their level of teaching responsibilities.

Finally, it implies that laboratories have the necessary equipment for the development of research and educational activities aligned with the needs of the profession (e.g. drug dosing software available).

Pharmacy Areas of Practice and Pharmacy Workforce

In Portugal, once pharmacy students finalize their master's degree, they may register with the regulatory professional body, the Portuguese Pharmaceutical Society (PPS). This is not compulsory for all areas of practice, but only for those that deliver the "pharmaceutical act", defined according to the Statute of the Pharmaceutical Society, most recently updated in 2015 (Law 131/2015).

According to this diploma, the pharmaceutical act comprises various activities: development and preparation of pharmaceutical forms; registry, production and quality control of medicines for human and veterinary use and medical devices; storing, conservation, and wholesale distribution; preparation, control, selection, and medicines dispensing in community, hospital and any other private or public pharmacies; preparation of anti-septic solutions and intravenous mixtures; interpretation and validation of medical prescriptions; information provision to patients and other healthcare professionals; monitoring medicines use and pharmacovigilance; drug monitoring, including pharmacokinetics determination and establishment of individualized therapeutic regime plans; collection of biologic samples, execution and interpretation of clinical analysis and determination of serum levels; execution, interpretation and validation of toxicological, hydrologic and bromatological analysis.

According to the International Pharmaceutical Federation (FIP), most pharmacists work in community pharmacies, as reported by the PPS (International Pharmaceutical Federation, 2015) (Ordem dos Farmacêuticos, 2018). Nonetheless, masters in pharmaceutical sciences practicing in other areas may, if they wish and see any benefit, also register, in which case they become pharmacists.

The professional workforce has been progressively growing, also in line with the growing number of faculties. The most recent data from the PPS refer to 2017 and indicate there are 14,423 active pharmacists. Most of these (59%) will practice in community pharmacy, followed by hospital pharmacy (9%), pharmaceutical industry (6%), pathology laboratories (5%), wholesaling (4%), education (2%) and research (1%) (Ordem dos Farmacêuticos, 2018).

One should consider that these data originate from the PPS, so under-representation from areas of practice beyond community and hospital pharmacy is likely to exist. The trend for professional workforce increase is consistent across almost all OECD countries. Data comparing the number of pharmacists per capita from 2000 to 2015 highlights Portugal as one of the four countries with the most rapid increase (OECD, 2017).

Ensuring the Competence of Pharmacists

The MSc degree teaches pharmacists to think and to become prepared to solve practical issues that may arise in the course of their professional activities. However, specific post-graduate education may be needed to gain knowledge, skills, and attitudes for an area of practice. Most faculties offer post-graduate programs, either in the format of seminars, short-courses, or even medium to long-term courses leading to an additional degree (second cycle MSc or Ph.D.). Other types of post-graduate education may also be offered by various entities outside the university. So, it is imperative for the profession to ensure these entities provide quality education.

The PPS was one of the pioneer structures at the international level to develop compulsory continuous professional development (CPD). CPD may be defined as the professional individual responsibility of pharmacists to constantly and systematically develop their knowledge, competences, and skills throughout their active life. This principle is in fact embedded into the ethical conduct of pharmacists in many countries and currently considered in the competency frameworks developed by various organizations, including the FIP, the European Association of Hospital Pharmacists, the American College of Clinical Pharmacists, to name a few.

The PPS Statute established by law states that pharmacists have the duty to promote and constantly update their knowledge by attending continuous development courses (Law 131/2015, 4th September).

The PPS model imposes that for the pharmacist to keep his license to practice, he/she needs to renew his/her knowledge through long-life learning. This model establishes 5-year cycles of evaluation, during which the pharmacist should make proof of having collected a total of 15 Credit units (Ordem dos Farmacêuticos, 2018). These units are attributed according to evidence of practice (2 credit units per year, up to a total of 10 credits) and evidence of attending courses (0.1 credit units per hour of learning or 0.15 if subject to evaluation). Teaching activities are also awarded credits (0.3 credit units per hour), which is consistent with pedagogical theories of valuing learning styles. On the other hand, unlike the previous regulations in place, participation in research activities is no longer valued, which may be a pitfall of the current model.

However, some authors argue that quantity is not necessarily quality so it is more important to measure the result of the learning activity than the hours of learning (Guskey TR, Unavailable date). This is the reason why learning activities having an evaluation are valued more than those not evaluated. Nonetheless, being able to answer a written test does not necessarily imply we can apply the knowledge acquired. For these reasons, some other countries have favored alternative methods of evaluation of learning activities.

The reflective model is one such example through which healthcare professionals are not required to send their certificates of attendance but are instead asked to submit a portfolio showing their reflections about what they learned and how they applied it to their practice. This is, of course, a much more time-consuming model of evaluation, both for the pharmacist under evaluation but also for the regulatory body making the assessment.

Another imperative to ensure up-to-date knowledge and competence in the various areas is to guide possible career pathways. A good and current example is the creation of a pharmaceutical career within the National Health Service (Pharmaceutical Residency), which will be headed at hospital pharmacists, clinical analysis and human genetics specialists, whose terms are being defined by law to ensure they have adequate theoretical and practical training during the phase of specialization following the university degree (Guidance on the Labour Law applicable to public health workers [Available in Portuguese: Normas com incidência nos trabalhadores com vínculo de emprego público, regulado pela lei geral do trabalho em funções públicas, aprovada em anexo à lei nº 35/2014], 2019).

Following the international trends, the Portuguese Pharmaceutical Society initiated work in the development of competency frameworks in 2014. These were focused on the professional areas of activity and aimed to identify and define the competencies required and those desired within each area of practice (Ordem dos Farmacêuticos, 2014). Four frameworks were then developed, including for hospital pharmacy, community pharmacy, pharmaceutical industry, and regulatory affairs. In the current year, a revised version of the regulation for the attribution of pharmaceutical competences has just been released (Ordem dos Farmacêuticos, 2019).

In addition to the competency frameworks, there are six areas of specialization approved in Portugal, including community pharmacy, clinical analysis, hospital pharmacy, pharmaceutical industry, regulatory affairs, and human genetics. The latest numbers available indicate there are in total 2684 specialist pharmacists in Portugal, so corresponding to 18.6% of the total registered pharmacists. Specialization is necessary for the pharmacist to be able to integrate one of the Boards of Pharmacy Practice and compulsory to be able to assume specific functions in practice, namely being technical director of a clinical analysis laboratory. This requirement is however not uniform, so to become technical director of a community pharmacy, it is not compulsory to have the specialist title, which may be considered an inconsistency of the regulatory system in place.

Unlike the CPD model previously explained, which heavily focuses on attending courses, becoming a specialist in any area demands specific regulations, including having relevant and documented experience in practice and obtain approval at the board of practice exam, which may be written or oral or both, according to the specific specialty area applied for. There is specific regulation in place defining in detail the demands for each of these specialty areas, which is embedded in the law (general regulation established by the Regulation 486/2018, and specific additional regulations for each area).

Importance of Specializations

As explained in the previous section, one main difference of the pathway leading to certification and specialization is the practical and on-site training. It is well established for many years that the ability to retain what we learn depends heavily on the learning experiences.

Around one week after having attended a lecture, for example, we will remember roughly 20% of what we heard. Conversely, one week after having undertaken such activity in a real-life context, we will retain 90% of the experience gained (Figure 1).

A second concept extremely relevant in the context of specialization is the conscious competence ladder, also known as the conscious competence matrix. This concept relates self-perception of our won ability to perform certain tasks and our true ability to execute them, so in other words, it relates conscience with competence.

The concept tells you that when you finalize your theoretical learning, often at the end of the university you are at the first stage or step of the ladder. At this stage, you truly believe you know it all, where in fact you have never had the opportunity (or had very little) to apply in practice your theory-based knowledge, implying you are in fact incompetent, although believing you are competent – this phase is named the unconscious incompetent.

You then start practicing and become progressively more aware of how little you know, which leads you to move into the second stage, *i.e.* the consciously incompetent.

As you progress in practice, you become more skilled in your daily tasks but it is still very much a process where you have to think before you act to make sure every action, every process is correctly delivered or implemented; this implies you are entering the third phase, which is the consciously competent phase.

Figure 1. The Cone of Learning
Source: (Northwest Center for Public Health Practice at the University of Washington School of Public Health, 2014)

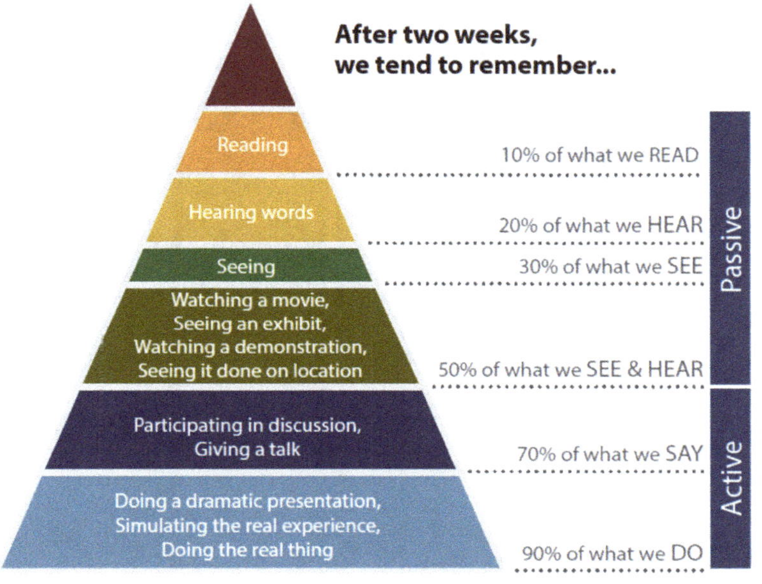

Finally, as you become even more experienced, you get to a stage where no longer you need to think about what you are doing, it becomes a natural process to do it well, so this implies you have entered the fourth and last step of the ladder, the unconsciously competent phase.

For all these reasons, the regulations guiding the acquisition of specialties are grounded in practice, and all assume to get to the last stage you need a minimum of three years.

ISSUES AND CONTROVERSIES

There are various reasons why we believe education is not totally adapted to the needs and demands of society and of employers in general. We present some of these sequentially, with no order, while arguing how they may be possibly solved.

Figure 2. The conscious competence matrix
Source: (Lyn Corno, 2015)

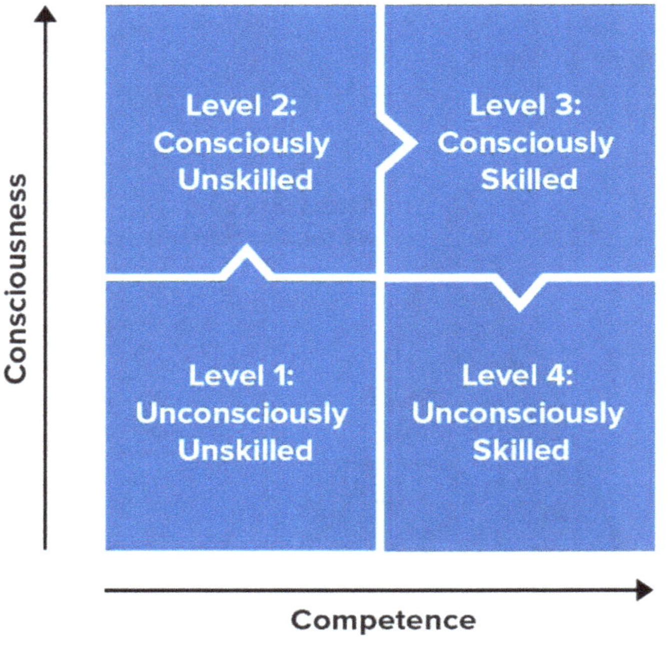

Challenges in Education

There are various challenges in pharmacy education, namely the maturity of students when they apply to a higher degree level, the innovation in teaching and evaluation methods, the infrastructures in place, the integration of the curriculum into practice, the lack of a patient-centered approach to teaching and isolation of degrees which aim to culminate in collaborative practices.

Maturity of Students

A person develops from childhood into adulthood in roughly 18 to 21 years, depending on the country's legal status. However, depending on the culture the person is brought up in, in more ancient and currently considered developing countries, children are treated as adults quite early, gaining the rights and duties to find their survival means quite early.

However, in industrialized countries, the trend is exactly the opposite. Children live with their overprotecting parents until very late, which leads to a level of immaturity that may be considered very relevant when it comes to choosing their degree at 17 or 18 years and their career path at 22 years of age.

This phenomenon calls for alternatives in terms of education that may either be modular, enabling students to direct their career as they progress through their maturity, or achieved by progressive integration into the profession, through which students have contact with different areas of their profession throughout the degree so that they can understand the usefulness of certain topics.

A possible approach is through what is called vertical learning, where the depth and the approach of what is taught evolve throughout the degree, but still contributing to solving the same problem. This is the approach taken at Monash University, where a core set of diseases (the most prevalent ones) were chosen and the course structure was rethought to provide solutions to tackle those diseases from a pharmaceutical perspective (Bruno-Tomé, 2018).

The Innovation of Teaching Methods and Infrastructures

The pharmacy profession has been changing in focus and demands for the various areas of practice, in Europe and globally (Martins, 2015).

Providing community pharmacy as an example, merely because it is still the most common area of practice, various regulatory changes have been implemented over the last decade in Portugal, impacting on service provision by community pharmacists. The first decree establishing the pharmaceutical services allowed in pharmacies was published in 2007 and more recently updated in 2018 (Ordinance 1429/2007; and Ordinance 97/2018).

Some of the services listed include pharmaceutical care, medication adherence, administration of vaccines, and screening tests for human immunodeficiency virus (HIV), hepatitis B and C (HCV and HBV), to name just a few. Looking at this restricted list, it becomes quite clear that none of the nine faculties provide students with the necessary education and training to be able to provide these services when registering to practice.

To simplify our arguments, we will focus on medication adherence, a quite straightforward service, but which desirably enables the student to become skilled at least with measurement methods and with enabling strategies.

Choosing simply one measurement method is often considered one of the most robust, we will take the example of the medication electronic monitoring systems (known as MEMS), where to our knowledge, no faculty uses these devices in teaching. Currently, there are more advanced and sophisticated methods, such as the Proteus system, recently approved by FDA, or even the older and most traditional measurements of drug biomarkers in urine or blood samples, again none of those used in practical teaching.

Regarding the enabling strategy, one of the most used in practice is the multicompartment aids system or dose dispensing aids (DAAs), mostly focusing on unintentional non-adherence, and secondly motivational interviewing, more directed at intentional non-adherence. To our knowledge, there are some courses supported using DAAs, albeit sporadic and not representative of teaching methods to support clinical pharmacy teaching in Portugal. Conversely, motivational interventions to enable medication adherence are not taught in faculty; hence not surprising that this service is hardly implemented in practice. This limitation is mostly associated with a lack of resources from academia, perhaps a lack of motivation from teachers, and certainly a lack of strategic vision that education should be aligned with practice.

However, the most controversial issue is when this lack of alignment arises from regulations in place, as it is the case of immunization. Some faculties have since 2007 restructured their curricula to prepare students for this new challenge of the profession. However, this simply makes them more prepared and competent for the challenges they will face in real life, but they will still have to undergo specific post-graduate training as the current regulations state that undergraduate education cannot be recognized by the professional body (Ordem dos Farmacêuticos, Direção Nacional, 2018). This, in our view, is a way to incentivize education not to align with practice demands. An opposite approach has been followed in Ireland for example, where following the uptake of this new service by pharmacists a two-stage process was followed: adaption of pharmacists already in practice (by offering specific courses to ensure competency); followed by the adaption of the undergraduate curriculum (by including the necessary topics, both theoretical and practical, in the syllabus, so that when students become pharmacists they are immediately fit for practice).

Contact with Patients Throughout the Degree

Following the national evaluation of pharmacy degrees conducted in Portugal during 2017/2018, it was finally documented what was perceived by many as a problem in most faculties. Most students will only see a real patient for the first time once they start their internship, which is planned to happen in the second semester of the fifth year.

There are obviously exceptions, where some faculties have specific topics allowing students to contact with patients in the course of an optional curricular unit, like hospital pharmacy. There are also some initiatives through which publicly open clinics within the university campus enable students to contact patients and gain some experience in dealing with the public. These are however only available from the fourth year onwards, which limits the applicability of the initiative and the contact period for the fortunate ones.

This is failing still in many European countries and which is not common to other health-related courses such as medicine, nursing, or dentistry where students can practice with real patients before finalizing their degree. The perception that students need to have earlier contacts to improve their skills has led some countries to renew their educational system, making it compulsory for students to progressively gain contact with the real world starting in the first year of university.

This is the case in Scotland, where students in initial years merely observe patient contact by shadowing professionals in the field, later interact directly with patients while constantly supervised by professionals, and in the final years become progressively more independent. It has been shown that this system is aligned with the conscious competence ladder previously introduced and shown to lead to better fitness for practice (MPharm in Pharmacy, 2019).

Interprofessional Collaboration

Another aspect that may be pointed out as an educational failure is the inability to integrate various health care professionals in teaching and learning. It has long been argued that if pharmacists, nurses, and physicians would interact as colleagues in some common curricular units during their degree, their future collaboration while becoming professionals would be much smoother and more successful.

However, most degrees in Portugal still fail to have teachers from these three professions working together or teaching students from these three courses together in the same classroom. Again, there are exceptions, mostly occurring in faculties that are integrated into hospital facilities, but these are unfortunately still a minority.

Distance from Practice

The lack of alignment between education and practice has been signaled in various areas and pharmacy is no exception. The European Students Association in collaboration with the European Association of Faculties of Pharmacy has launched a project in 2012 named the Methodology Booklet, which aims to collect pharmacy students and recent graduates' opinions about teaching methods, ultimately aiming to share these with educators.

The first report made available in 2018, pertaining to results obtained from 29 countries, including Portugal, suggested that some teaching methodologies beyond the traditional format are lacking and sometimes only made available through students' association initiatives rather than embedded in regular teaching (European Pharmacy Students Association, 2018). The most frequently reported form of teacher-student interaction was "the teacher talks, and the students listen", stated by 64% of respondents. The inability of education to adapt to new technologies seems to emerge from such report, where technologies for long-existing in other contexts are here presented as future, namely, streamline teaching, case simulations using virtual environments, online or smartphone apps enabling interaction, gaming as a learning technique, to name a few. In fact, aiming to answer this perceived problem, students proactively engaged in developing their own Lifelong Learning Platform (LLeaP), through which they use some of these techniques (e.g. gaming) to motivate learning.

Also, a report issued by McKinsey referring to a study exploring employers' perceptions of recent graduates suggested a low level of alignment between education and market needs (Mona Mourshed, 2012). This report suggests that even in years and countries facing high unemployment rates, which has never been the case for pharmacy, 31% of employers state to be unable to fill their vacancies because recent graduates do not have the necessary qualifications for the jobs. Aditionally, it was shown that the perceptions of teachers are quite different from employers; specifically questioned if they feel the education is appropriate for market needs, 74% of teachers answered positively, as opposed to only 35% of employers.

This data suggests that most educators probably do not practice outside academia, which may be natural given the most common situation is to have an exclusivity contract. In the UK, the concept of teacher-practitioner has long been embedded into the educational system, a measure aimed at ensuring professors articulate with practitioners, involving them in their curricular units, while practitioners bring real cases, current and up-to-date practices and infra-structures to class.

The Role of the Regulator

As previously explained, the Bologna Declaration establishes the number of ECTS comprised by the MSc in pharmaceutical sciences but it also states that there are core areas that need to be reflected in the course structure, and also in the ratio of professors with a given specific degree, for the courses to be recognized by the Ministry of Education and approved by law.

Table 1 summarizes the educational offer in Portugal in the nine institutions existing in 2019.

Analyzing this table, it seems the offer is quite similar across all faculties, exception made perhaps to the postgraduate offer. However, this table is merely showing the general trends and is not detailing the teaching methods used, the teaching environment, the proportion of practical training, to name a few.

A very good example is the teaching of clinical pharmacy, which may be delivered in various formats, all of them shown to have quite different impacts on competencies acquired by students. Purely expositive teaching is one possible format, practicing by solving theory-based clinical cases in a paper, practicing by solving real cases taken from practice (normally brought to faculty by teacher-practitioners), practicing by web-based simulation where the case (normally fictitious) may take different formats depending on the interaction made with the student, or practicing in a real-life scenario (normally hospital-based).

Table 1. Main features in the MSC in Pharmaceutical in Portugal

Faculties	ECTS Conferred MSc	Area With the Strongest Component	Proportion of Employed Graduates	Post-graduate Offer	Particularities
Institution 1	300	Pharmaceutical Sciences	94.8%	6 MSc; 1 PG; 1 PhD	• Various international partners. • Unique center for monitoring drug-herbal interactions.
Institution 2	300	Pharmaceutical Sciences	99.4%	7 MSc; 3 PG; 5 PhD	• Various partnerships with other faculties for Ph.D.
Institution 3	300	Health Sciences	95.0%	6 PhD	• Various partnerships with other faculties for Ph.D.
Institution 4	300	Biology and Biochemistry	94.9%	3 MSc;	• Compulsory internships throughout the degree in various areas.
Institution 5	300	Pharmaceutical Sciences	95.0%	4 MSc; 14 PG	• Summer internships throughout the degree in various areas.
Institution 6	300	Pharmaceutical Sciences	98.1%	1 MSc; 1 PhD	• Sole institution with growing number of students
Institution 7	300	Pharmaceutical Sciences	95.7%	10 PG; 1 PhD	• Teacher practitioner concept (integrated with the local community). • Interprofessional collaboration in teaching (e.g. clinical cases).
Institution 8	300	Pharmaceutical Sciences	Not Available		• Has own hospital to ensure internships.
Institution 9	300	Pharmaceutical Sciences	95.0%	1 MSc; 1 PhD	• International partnerships for PhD. Teaching organized in trimesters.

This shows us then when analyzing course content merely by analyzing the decrees published; we have absolutely no information on the quality of education provided. It also shows that imposing rules per se does not solve problems.

THE PORTUGUESE EDUCATION AND PRACTICE PLATFORM (EPP)

The Education & Practice Platform (EPP) is an entity developed within the PPS, following the indications announced by the Board of Directors on the mandate 2016-2019, to meet the common interests of academia and practitioners. This implies that the EPP acts in two parallel fields of action: on the academic side, aiming to influence the innovation in teaching methods; and on the professional side, aiming to collect information about key competencies for each practice area that needs to be ensured through life-long learning to have a competent pharmaceutical workforce.

Development was initiated by identifying the characteristics of representatives, coordinators, and the short and long-term aims of EPP. The EPP includes one representative from each of the nine pharmacy faculties and one representative from the six Councils of Specialty Boards of Practice (CSBP).

The EPP's mission, vision, and values were then set by the steering group created during a face-to-face meeting. Its mission is to evaluate the quality and adequacy of education from the perspective of professional integration; to foster quality development in teaching practices with recognition for autonomy in freedom to teach and to learn.

Its vision is the alignment of education and practice with the PPS' statutes to ensure validation of the competences defined for each practice area and compliance with the guidance from international organizations. Its values were defined as "strong links between academia and the profession"; "adequacy to societal demands"; "adequacy of teaching to the new areas of the profession"; and "recognition of the existing human capital".

During the initial meeting of the EPP, a brainstorming activity with all involved parties was organized to share concerns and interests and to identify a common path. Based on the results of this initial activity, a one-year plan was drawn. This plan included the development of two workshops tackling two of the major concerns of educators and practitioners: teaching methods and internships' organization. Both activities were organized as a two-fold activity, where the first used a more expositive approach providing the basic concepts and possible alternatives, and the second was organized in a more practical manner aiming to foster self-reflection from all involved.

To mark the launch of the EPP, we created a logo representing a flower that will blossom and become professional. This flower is composed of nine petals, five in green, and four in white representing the two groups of public and private institutions in Portugal (Figure 3).

Figure 3. Logo of the Education and Practice Platform

How Can EPP Contribute to Align Education and Practice?

Involvement in International Events

During the initial brainstorming activity, there was a perceived need for greater involvement of academia in international events focusing on education. The EEP was perceived as a possible means for identification, prioritizing of events and dissemination of selected ones, whilst encouraging active participation.

Since the EPP was initiated, the representation in international events has increased. To name a few, an oral communication was presented at FIP summarizing the work here described with greater detail and, in addition, a poster was presented at the Innovations in Pharmacy Congress held to celebrate the 100 years of the University of Salamanca. In 2018/2019, the EPP participated in an international study developed by the European Society of Clinical Pharmacy (ESCP), through which information on the weight of clinical pharmacy-related topics in pre-graduate education in all institutions was provided (Table 2).

Table 2. Clinical pharmacy component of Pharmaceutical Sciences MSc degrees in Portugal

Institution	# Semesters	# Contact Hours / Semester	# ECTS/ Semester	% Practical Teaching
1	3	56	5	73
2	1	60	5	43
3	2	60	4	33
4	2	112	9	68
5	1	60	5	50
6	3	52	5	67
7	2	49	4	60
8	1	75	6	60
9	1	52	4	50

Note: Optional topics were excluded from this analysis; only topics within the scope of clinical pharmacy, as defined by ESCP, were considered, which means that e.g. pharmacology and pharmacotherapy are not included.

Answering Global Requests

In line with the limited involvement in international events, most EEP representatives were unaware of global advances in pharmacy education and as such the EPP was committed to regularly update all representatives on relevant initiatives, namely to be used as a liaison between National academia and international organizations with a special focus on education, such as the FIPEd, the European Society of Clinical Pharmacy Education Committee (ESCP EdComm), the European Association of Faculties of Pharmacy (EAFP), to name a few; while also being involved with pharmacy students international organization, such as the European Pharmaceutical Students' Association (EPSA) or the International Pharmacy Students' Federation (IPSF).

The first activity within this domain developed by the EPP was the adaption of the Workforce Development Goals (WDGs), issued by FIP, to Portuguese, once permission was officially granted. A summary brochure with the WDGs was distributed in the National Congress of Pharmacists held in October 2017 to all participants (n=1500). This brochure served various purposes: 1) to introduce the EPP and explain its intention; 2) to present the WDGs developed by FIP; 3) to map the national situation in 2017.

The details of the workforce development Goals are presented in chapter 2. Once the Report "Transforming Pharmacy and Pharmaceutical Sciences Education in the Context of Workforce Development" was issued in Portuguese by the FIP, the EPP also ensured all members were made aware of it (Federação Internacional Farmacêutica (FIP), 2017). Later, as the EPP started to become more widespread, it became responsible for providing information to external bodies about education in pharmaceutical sciences in Portugal.

As such, the EPP has collaborated in two surveys providing information about the evolution of meeting the WDG (developed by FIP) and on education and practice in clinical pharmacy (developed by the ESCP).

Answering National Needs

Although there is a national framework for education in pharmaceutical sciences publicly announcing the main features of the degree, the differences in specific topics offered, organization of teaching activities, internships, MSc theses, and post-graduate education were unmapped.

As such, one major feature of the EPP in all activities developed has been sharing and benchmarking, adopting a constructive criticism approach. This means in fact that all participants were encouraged to openly share their curricular details, including not only the main features published in official documents, but also the internal working procedures, including class organization, teaching methods, materials, facilities, and by working in this climate, all opened up their own "box of Pandora", gaining space for others to share their own flaws, whilst presenting also different approaches, some of which could be used as ideas to be adapted to improve their weakest points.

As explained earlier, CPD is mandatory in Portugal. The PPS is the responsible body for attributing ECTS according to the demands of the course. However, various entities may offer CPD to practicing pharmacists. It was considered to be in the best interest of the regulatory body, of the practicing pharmacists and of the potential providers of CPD, to establish a partnership protocol between the PPS and the nine institutions for the provision of post-graduate education in strategic areas. These areas will be annually identified by the Councils of Specialty Boards of Practice and conveyed to academia so that they may organize consortia between different schools, eventually including also other professionals, to increase the quality and the diversity of CPD, while ensuring geographical distribution.

Workshop Activities

The first workshop focused on teaching models and the adaption of the curricula to become practice-centered and student-centered.

An example from the University of Monash was presented (Bruno-Tomé, 2018), where vertical teaching was adopted so that all the topics in the curriculum may interact, making their utility for practice evident (Postma TC, 2017). The methodology booklet produced by EPSA was also presented, where students shared their views on the current educational model while clearly criticizing the expositive approach and the lack of alignment with practice.

Following these two activities, participants were mixed, creating groups of faculty members from different institutions and practitioners and were asked to select one topic area and think which feasible changes they could implement to better tailor their teaching to modern methods and also to students' expressed desires.

The second workshop focused on the mandatory final unit which comprises internships in a community or hospital pharmacy, as imposed by the European Pharmaceutical Sciences Graduation Directive, where all faculty members shared their internship plan, how it was organized, evaluated and monitored. Subsequently, practitioners shared their experiences and concerns when confronted with students from different institutions in their practice, either in the community or in the hospital. In this event, apart from the regular six representatives of the CSBP, where two of them gave their testimony about the concerned areas (community and hospital), representatives from the two pharmacy owners associations and the Portuguese association of hospital pharmacists were also present.

Finally, the experience from students was also shared, while suggesting possible new solutions for a unified and improved integration into the profession.

The third workshop followed the discussions on internships and was organized in a similar format but focusing on the internship in hospital pharmacy. As a supplementary activity aiming to tackle another failure in the current educational system, representatives from patient advocacy organizations were invited to share their experiences of working collaboratively with academia and reach agreement on possible ways of collaborating also with the pharmacy faculties.

Various collaborative models identified which may be taken up in the future include their inclusion in teaching some modules within varied curricular units throughout the degree (e.g. person-centered pharmaceutical care and shared decision making), collaboration in the identification of topics or the final thesis, or even co-supervision, and involvement also in the internships.

Other features emerging included the insertion of patient representatives in the strategic units of faculties, involvement in juries for varying levels of education, and planning and implementation of conferences headed at students or professionals.

DISCUSSION AND FUTURE DIRECTIONS OF EPP

To bring academics to the PPS was one aim of the EPP, which has been clearly achieved with the regular meetings organized. Additionally, we intended to contribute to greater proximity between pharmacists' under and post-graduation education and professional capacities.

This institutional program launched by the PPS in collaboration with all the academic partners for pharmacists' education in Portugal and with the representatives of the employers of the various areas of practice is unique and enabled greater awareness of academics about current practice while also opening current educational trends to practitioners.

Sitting practitioners from different areas together with academics to share their views and seek common solutions to achieve a stronger workforce is only a starting point. To achieve clear cut results, much work is still to be developed.

The program was developed under the umbrella of the PPS. This is found to be a major strength as it enabled the commitment from all the Boards of Practice, obviously of utmost importance for sharing framework practices and current and future healthcare system needs that may be useful to incorporate in curriculum design.

The fact that Portugal is a small country might have helped to be able to involve all nine faculties. Nonetheless, our experience tells us that this opportunity for frequent gathering to discuss common interests contributed to teambuilding, where academia is a unique team rather than nine teams, as we all are interested in contributing to the same: a better pharmacist for the future. Furthermore, the option for a stepwise approach enabled building a shared vision, and a common path to meet the needs of the future. The regular discussion of practices, considering international and national experiences, standards, and guidelines is an additional strength of the project itself.

Many of the educational mismatches with practice identified so far are perhaps not new. However, the fact that they were identified by all, using an open fora process, where everyone's views are considered equal, including teachers, students and practitioners, is crucial for assuming shared commitments for change.

As an example, we cite the need for more clinical pharmacy training, a shared concern by academia, hospital pharmacist and community pharmacists. The need to innovate in clinical pharmacy has long been debated and the creation of practice-partnerships has been proposed as a possible solution, whilst recognizing the difficulties of putting this idea into practice sometimes due to cultural or contextual barriers (Gubbins PO, 2014).

Data gathered comparing our nine faculties have highlighted the diversity in clinical pharmacy, not only in terms of quantitative weight in the curricular structure but also in terms of practical teaching methods adopted. Certainly, there are limitations to the analysis shown, namely the fact that optional topics have been ignored and some faculties have a strong offer in clinical pharmacy provided by such topics (e.g. hospital pharmacy). There is also the possibility of misclassification, as some topics have names that may or not fit into the definition of clinical pharmacy (e.g. pharmacy practice; pharmacy laboratory).

Nonetheless, we believe such biases have been equally distributed and the purpose of the exercise was mostly to verify existing diversity. Certainly, clinical pharmacy is just one possible area, and if we would focus on another, results could eventually be quite different. Currently, we are all aware of contextual differences between our faculties but will focus on identifying tailored solutions that may result in shared learning outcomes.

Despite its merits, this initiative has also some limitations worth acknowledging. The fact that it is not a research project with a specific timeline and very clear-cut indicators makes implementation more difficult and difficult to monitor. Academics and practitioners have often different views, making debates challenging, which is not a limitation per se but may hinder the progress of changes intended. Perhaps the most important limitation, which is still potential, and we hope to be able to overcome it, is the inability to ensure this initiative will be sustained in future PPS' mandates. The way we anticipate being able to solve this is by giving the EPP free wings to be able to fly independently in the future, maintaining the ability to align education and practice for the sake of a more qualified pharmaceutical workforce, with or without political support.

CONCLUSION

The scope of practice of pharmacists has been changing worldwide (Costa FA, 2019) (Imfeld-Isenegger, 2019) (Costa F, 2017). Education needs to keep up the pace and adapt accordingly. Throughout this chapter, we have reviewed the evolution of pharmacy education in Portugal, expressed mostly personal views of the current status of education, highlighting the major pitfalls according to our perception.

We then describe the creation of an Education and Practice Platform, which certainly will not solve all the identified limitations in the educational model, but hopeful will modestly contribute to a better alignment between education and practice and thus contribute to a more skilled and competent pharmaceutical workforce that may best meet the needs of our society.

REFERENCES

Bruno-Tomé, A. (2018). *Teaching methodologies: the experience from Monash University*. Lisboa, Portugal: Academic Press.

Costa, F., Scullin, C., Al-Anni, G., Hawwa, A., McElnay, J., Hersberger, K., & Westerlund, T. (2017). Provision of pharmaceutical care by community pharmacists across Europe: Is it developing and spreading? *Journal of Evaluation in Clinical Practice*, *23*(6), 1336–1347.

Costa, F.A., Lee, V., Tous, S., Papastergiou, J., Neubeck, L., Freedman, B., & Antoniou, S. (2019). Awareness campaigns of Atrial Fibrillation as an opportunity for early detection by pharmacists- an international cross-sectional study. *Journal of Thrombosis and Thrombolysis*. . doi:10.100711239-019-02000-x

dos Farmacêuticos, O. (2014). *Model for the Attribution of Pharmaceutical Competences and Specialties*. Obtido em 16 de 2 de 2019, de www.ordemfarmaceuticos.pt

dos Farmacêuticos, O. (2018). *Farmacêuticos em números*. Obtido em 23 de 11 de 2019, de https://www.ordemfarmaceuticos.pt/pt/numeros/

dos Farmacêuticos, O. (2018). *Ordem dos Farmacêuticos*. Obtido em 8 de 11 de 2019, de Regulamento interno de qualificação.: https://www.ordemfarmaceuticos.pt/fotos/documentos/regulamento_interno_de_qualificacao_versao_final_10071147805c1a3a94b2e41.pdf

dos Farmacêuticos, O. (2019). *Regulation for the Attribution of Pharmaceutical Competences*. Obtido de www.ordemfarmaceuticos.pt

dos Farmacêuticos, O., & Nacional, D. (2018). Reconhecimento de Formação de Farmacêuticos. Administração de vacinas e medicamentos injectáveis em farmácia comunitária.

European Pharmacy Students Association. (2018). *Methodology Booklet*. European Commission.

Federação Internacional Farmacêutica (FIP). (2017). *Transformar a formação e educação em farmácia e ciências farmacêuticas no contexto da força laboral farmacêutica*. Obtido em 18 de 2 de 2019, de https://fip.org/files/fip/PharmacyEducation/FIPEd_Nanjing_Report_2017_PT.pdf

Gubbins, P. O. M. S. (2014). Innovation in clinical pharmacy practice and opportunities for academic—practice partnership. *Pharmacotherapy, 34*(5), 45-54. http://bte.gep.msess.gov.pt/separatas/sep33_2019.pdf

Guskey, T.R. (n.d.). *Evaluating professional development*. University of Kentucky.

Imfeld-Isenegger, T. L., Soares, I. B., & Hersberger, K. E. (2019). Pharmacist-led medication review procedures: a survey across Europe. Research in Social and Administrative Pharmacy. doi:10.1016/j.saph

International Pharmaceutical Federation. (2015). *Global trends shaping pharmacy - Regulatory Frameworks, Distribution of Medicines and Professional Services, 2013-2015*. Author.

Lyn Corno, E. M. (2015). *Handbook of Educational Psychology*. Routledge. doi:10.4324/9781315688244

Martins, S., van Mil, J. W. F., & Costa, F. A. (2015). The Organizational Framework of Community Pharmacies in Europe. *International Journal of Clinical Pharmacy, 37*(5), 896–905. doi:10.100711096-015-0140-1 PMID:26017399

Mona Mourshed, D. F. (2012). *Education to Employment: Designing a system that works*. McKinsey Center for Government.

MPharm in Pharmacy. (2019). Obtido de University of Strathclyde, Scotland: https://www.strath.ac.uk/courses/undergraduate/pharmacy/

Northwest Center for Public Health Practice at the University of Washington School of Public Health. (2014). *Effective Adult Learning. A toolkit for teaching adults*. Robert Wood Johnson Foundation.

OECD. (2017). *Health at a Glance: Pharmaceutical Sector*. OECD.

Postma, T. C., & White, J. G. (2017). Students' perceptions of vertical and horizontal integration in a discipline-based dental school? *European Journal of Dental Education*, *21*(2), 101–107. doi:10.1111/eje.12186 PMID:26801357

Conclusion

Stepwise approach into a future, that is already with us...

The authors have to be congratulated for giving a first step in the right direction. That moment certainly needs now stronger support and deeper mobilization of Universities in the coming years ahead. It is the first time that we see academics and professionals together looking into pedagogic aspects, their limitations, some solutions, aiming to improve the education and training of future pharmacists. Today, they just touched the surface, but as we all know, the first step is always the one facing more resistance and the one facing more uncertainty. Honor to their courage and commitment.

Undergraduate training in Pharmaceutical Sciences, in Portugal as in other European Union countries, integrates the basic set of requirements for being a registered Pharmacist, embedded both in the Law and in a (challenged) traditional model for professional practice. Meanwhile, the healthcare sector is currently going through a profound transformation, in its processes and technologies, but also facing new societal challenges from groups and individuals. People are now more demanding for integrated and personalized health care responses and are also more conscious of their citizenship rights, in their communities and globally (*civitas maxima*).

Data analytics, cybersecurity and relevant aspects of quality of data integration, modeling and use of AI (mostly ML or deep machine learning) as well as virtual reality (VR) environments, all suitable for clinical training, can also be used in order to have more efficient interventions in the health care sector. Today they are challenging both undergraduate *curricula* but also the role of Universities and their inherent responsibilities, facing the needs of undergraduate training looking to the days of today and tomorrow, not those of yesterday.

Here we have to say (without any hesitation), that today's Universities are being highly challenged. Mostly because of their adherence to past practices and slow path of change, in pedagogic solutions and teaching instruments/tools, but also because their teaching staff is not seldom outdated and divorced from healthcare innovation, unable to use such modern instruments.

Schools of Pharmacy need to be fully integrated into University Academic Hospital Centres as already happens with Medical and Nursing Schools. This will lead to improved undergraduate training with a higher proportion of clinical training, but also integrating internships and post-graduated training within integrated health care training teams. Pharmacists are now integrated into a complex health care setting, within growing networks of healthcare professionals. As we move forward, that reality should be prepared within higher education, earlier in their undergraduate training.

The most important question for European Schools of Pharmacy is to move from a "medicines-centric" model to a "clinical-centered" model, that certainly needs strong competences in medicines research, development and use, but also in a set of competences and professional skills, in the use and integration of a diverse array of health technologies.

In general, a great number of European schools need also to learn lessons from our US colleagues and other regions in the world. PharmD *curricula* promote a more suitable clinically-oriented model of training, without losing the backbone of traditional "pharmaceutical knowledge". Integration between undergraduates and internships, promoting a wider array of clinically-oriented competences and knowledge, is essential to ensure an updated vision of pharmacist's role in the coming years.

Pharmacists are involved, more and more, in an environment with multiple layers of integration between diverse basic and applied sciences, certainly within the context of healthcare but also clearly centered on people and their health needs. Not only patients and citizens should be at the center of healthcare, as well as those frequently excluded from our societies and currently also threatened by global public health challenges. In fact, humanitarian crisis all along the Mediterranean and other European frontiers, during the last decade (and with a peak in 2015), showed how important it is also to consider the rights of those (migrants and refugees) that are not yet European citizens, but already within our borders and within our communities. Promoting the understanding of such complex societal phenomena has to be also a role for Universities that wish to train pharmacists that are engaged in societal impact, not aside from important societal issues.

Additive and distributed manufacturing technologies in an individualized care setting will certainly bring back the proximity role that pharmacists had already, both in compounding and patient counseling, delivering specific personalized solutions. Meanwhile, better knowledge and ability to promote integration and interpretation of vast and complex sets of data will also allow pharmacists to bring to the forefront of healthcare a hopeful generation of real-world evidence, with a transformational impact in healthcare.

Conclusion

Clinical Pharmacy, traditionally stronger within the Hospital setting, needs to be at the forefront of community pharmacists' role and their professional behavior. Similarly, deeper knowledge and use of advanced analytical tools and modeling skills will allow for Pharmacoepidemiology to reinforce both Clinical Pharmacy and a new role for Pharmacists in Public Health and Health Policies.

How we will prepare, hopefully, better and better, our current students to face the challenges of a global world — whose crisis are no longer compartmentalized in geographic terms — will deliver a societal-centered role for pharmacists or, in the opposite direction, a road to the decadence of pharmacists societal role.

As a consequence, deeper integration between basic and applied sciences, using highly innovative technologies and better training in ethics and social sciences, will shape the competences of the pharmacists, that are required to have again an increased role and impact in the future of society and also impacting the life of each and every one of us.

Rogério Sá Gaspar
Faculty of Pharmacy, Institute for Bioengineering and Biosciences, Instituto Superior Técnico, University of Lisbon, Portugal

Rogério Sá Gaspar *is a Full Professor at FFUL, Faculdade de Farmácia & Researcher at the Institute for Bioengineering and Biosciences from Instituto Superior Técnico, both at the Universidade de Lisboa.*

Compilation of References

Aburahma, M. H., & Mohamed, H. M. (2015). Educational games as a teaching tool in pharmacy curriculum. American Journal of Pharmaceutical Education. doi:10.5688/ajpe79459

Acesso ao Ensino Superior 2020 - Índices de Cursos (por curso e instituição). (n.d.). Retrieved September 30, 2020, from https://www.dges.gov.pt/guias/indcurso.asp?curso=9494

Adamo, J. E., Wilhelm, E. E., & Steele, S. J. (2015). Advancing a Vision for Regulatory Science Training. *Clinical and Translational Science*, *8*(5), 615–618. Advance online publication. doi:10.1111/cts.12298 PMID:26083660

Akdeniz, C. (2016). *Learning and Teaching: Theories, Approaches and Models* (2nd ed.). Çözüm Eğitim Yayıncılık.

ALA Presidential Committee on Information Literacy. (1989). *Final Report: American Library Association*. Author.

AlHaqwi, A. I., Kuntze, J., & van der Molen, H. T. (2014). Development of the clinical learning evaluation questionnaire for undergraduate clinical education: Factor structure, validity, and reliability study. *BMC Medical Education*, *14*(1), 44. doi:10.1186/1472-6920-14-44 PMID:24592913

Almeman, A. A., & Alrebish, S. A. (2018). Teaching Strategies Used in Pharmacy. In *Pharmacy Education in the Twenty First Century and Beyond* (pp. 125–145). Elsevier., doi:10.1016/B978-0-12-811909-9.00010-1

Alper, B. S., Hand, J. A., Elliott, S. G., Kinkade, S., Hauan, M. J., Onion, D. K., & Sklar, B. M. (2004). How much effort is needed to keep up with the literature relevant for primary care? *Journal of the Medical Library Association: JMLA*, *92*(4), 429–437. PMID:15494758

Alt, D. (2015). Assessing the contribution of a constructivist learning environment to academic self-efficacy in higher education. *Learning Environments Research*, *18*(1), 47–67. doi:10.100710984-015-9174-5

Altman, R. B., Khuri, N., Salit, M., & Giacomini, K. M. (2015). Unmet needs: Research helps regulators do their jobs. Science Translational Medicine. doi:10.1126citranslmed.aac4369

American College of Clinical Pharmacy. (2008). The definition of clinical pharmacy. *Pharmacotherapy*, 816–817. PMID:18503408

American Pharmacists Association. (2007). *Drug Information Handbook* (15th ed.). Lexi-Comp Inc.

Amerson, A. B., & Wallingford, D. M. (1983). Twenty years' experience with drug information centers. *American Journal of Hospital Pharmacy*, *40*(7), 1172–1178. doi:10.1093/ajhp/40.7.1172 PMID:6881155

Amundstuen Reppe, L., Spigset, O., & Schjott, J. (2016). Drug Information Services Today: Current Role and Future Perspectives in Rational Drug Therapy. *Clinical Therapeutics*, *38*(2), 414–421. doi:10.1016/j.clinthera.2015.12.019 PMID:26831829

Anderson, C., Bates, I., Beck, D., Brock, T., Futter, B., Mercer, H., … Yonemura, A. (2008). The WHO UNESCO FIP Pharmacy Education Taskforce: Enabling concerted and collective global action. *American Journal of Pharmaceutical Education*. doi:10.5688/aj7206127

Anderson, C., Bates, I., Beck, D., Brock, T. P., Futter, B., Mercer, H., Rouse, M., Whitmarsh, S., Wuliji, T., & Yonemura, A. (2009). The WHO UNESCO FIP Pharmacy Education Taskforce. *Human Resources for Health*, *7*(1), 45. Advance online publication. doi:10.1186/1478-4491-7-45 PMID:19500351

Andiwatir, A., & Betan, Y. (2019). Letter to the Editor: Evidence-based practice for nursing profession: Barriers and teaching strategies solutions. Int J Nurs Sci, 6(1), 123-124. doi:10.1016/j.ijnss.2018.11.009

Antunes, J. L. (2012). A Nova Medicina. (F. F. M. dos Santos, Ed.). Lisboa: Editores, Relógio D'Agua.

APIFARMA. (2019). *Ensaios clínicos em Portugal*. www.pwc.pt/s&cfa

Applin, H., Williams, B., Day, R., & Buro, K. (2011). A comparison of competencies between problem-based learning and non-problem-based graduate nurses. *Nurse Education Today*, *31*(2), 129–134. doi:10.1016/j.nedt.2010.05.003 PMID:20817332

APREFAR - APREFAR - Associação dos Profissionais de Registos e Regulamentação Farmacêutica. (n.d.). Retrieved October 1, 2020, from https://www.aprefar.pt/conteudos/?page=aprefar

Aromataris, E., & Munn, Z. (Eds.). (2017). *Joanna Briggs Institute Reviewer's Manual*. The Joanna Briggs Institute. Available from https://reviewersmanual.joannabriggs.org/

Asikainen, H. (2014). *Successful learning and studying in biosciences*. University of Helsinky.

Augustin, M. (2014). How to learn effectively in medical school: Test yourself, learn actively, and repeat in intervals. *The Yale Journal of Biology and Medicine*, *87*(2), 207–212. PMID:24910566

Ausubel, D. (1963). *The psychology of meaningful verbal learning*. University Press.

Azer, S. A., Guerrero, A. P., & Walsh, A. (2013). Enhancing learning approaches: Practical tips for students and teachers. *Medical Teacher*, *35*(6), 433–443. doi:10.3109/0142159X.2013.775413 PMID:23496121

Babar, Z. U. D., Kousar, R., Murtaza, G., Azhar, S., Khan, S. A., & Curley, L. (2018). Randomized controlled trials covering pharmaceutical care and medicines management: A systematic review of literature. *Research in Social & Administrative Pharmacy*. Advance online publication. doi:10.1016/j.sapharm.2017.06.008 PMID:28651923

Bach, A., & Goad, J. (2015). The role of community pharmacy-based vaccination in the USA: Current practice and future directions. *Integrated Pharmacy Research & Practice*. Advance online publication. doi:10.2147/iprp.s63822 PMID:29354521

Badyal, D. K., & Singh, T. (2017). Learning Theories: The Basics to Learn in Medical Education. *International Journal of Applied & Basic Medical Research*, *7*(5, Suppl 1), S1–S3. doi:10.4103/ijabmr.IJABMR_385_17 PMID:29344448

Balardim, G. (2020). *Metodologias de ensino: confira 10 das mais usadas nas escolas*. https://www.clipescola.com/metodologias-de-ensino-confira/

Balshem, H., Helfand, M., Schunemann, H. J., Oxman, A. D., Kunz, R., Brozek, J., ... Guyatt, G. H. (2011). GRADE guidelines: 3. Rating the quality of evidence. *Journal of Clinical Epidemiology*, *64*(4), 401–406. doi:10.1016/j.jclinepi.2010.07.015 PMID:21208779

Bansback, N., Keystone, E., O'Dell, J., Phibbs, C. S., Hannagan, K., Brophy, M., & Anis, A. (2015). Making smart investment decisions in clinical research. *Trials*, *16*(1), 590. doi:10.118613063-015-1123-1 PMID:26712327

Beck, R. J. (1980). Drug information program builds skills. *American Pharmacy*, *NS20*(1), 54. doi:10.1016/S0160-3450(15)32924-X PMID:7369124

Beecher Martins, C., & Soares, M. (2019). Visual Literacy Applied to Film Still Analysis in Medical Training. In Present 40th APEAA (pp. 1–11). Academic Press.

Belia, D. (2013). Traditional Teaching Methods Vs. Teaching Through The Application Of Information And Communication Technologies In The Accounting Field: Quo Vadis? *European Scientific Journal*, *9*(28).

Berland, G. K., Elliott, M. N., Morales, L. S., Algazy, J. I., Kravitz, R. L., Broder, M. S., Kanouse, D. E., Muñoz, J. A., Puyol, J.-A., Lara, M., Watkins, K. E., Yang, H., & McGlynn, E. A. (2001). Health information on the Internet: Accessibility, quality, and readability in English and Spanish. *Journal of the American Medical Association*, *285*(20), 2612–2621. doi:10.1001/jama.285.20.2612 PMID:11368735

Bernknopf, A. C., Karpinski, J. P., McKeever, A. L., Peak, A. S., Smith, K. M., Smith, W. D., Timpe, E. M., & Ward, K. E. (2009). Drug information: From education to practice. *Pharmacotherapy*, *29*(3), 331–346. doi:10.1592/phco.29.3.331 PMID:19249951

Bisrat, H., Abel, B., Salome, W., Michael, M., & Sade, H. (2018). Development of a New Innovative Teaching Method Using a Comprehensive Approach: A Survey of Students' Opinion. *Biomedical Journal of Scientific & Technical Research*, *3*(4).

Bleakley. (Ed.). (2020). *Routledge Handbook of the Medical Humanities*. Routledge.

Bollela, V. R., Senger, M. H., Tourinho, F. S. V, & Amaral, E. (2014). Aprendizagem baseada em equipes: da teoria à prática. *Medicina (Ribeirão Preto)*, *47*(3), 293–300.

Bonal, J. (1988). *The Clinical Pharmacist: Education Document*. European Society of Clinical Pharmacy.

Bowen, R. S. (2017). *Understanding by Design*. Vanderbilt University Center for Teaching. Retrieved from https://cft.vanderbilt.edu/understanding-by-design/

Brazeau, G. A., Meyer, S. M., Belsey, M., Bednarczyk, E. M., Bilic, S., Bullock, J., DeLander, G. E., Fiese, E. F., Giroux, S. L., McNatty, D., Nemire, R., Prescott, W. A. Jr, & Traynor, A. P. (2009). Preparing pharmacy graduates for traditional and emerging career opportunities. *American Journal of Pharmaceutical Education*, *73*(8), 157. doi:10.5688/aj7308157 PMID:20221350

Brett-MacLean, P. J., Cave, M. T., Yiu, V., Kelner, D., & Ross, D. J. (2010). Film as a means to introduce narrative reflective practice in medicine and dentistry: A beginning story presented in three parts. *Reflective Practice*, *11*(4), 499–516. doi:10.1080/14623943.2010.505713

Brito, A., Simões, A., Costa, F. A., & Alcobia, A. (2016). Revisão e reconciliação terapêutica em hospitalização domiciliária. *IX Congresso Nacional da APFH (Associação Portuguesa de Farmácia Hospitalar): Segurança & Inovação–Pilares do Futuro.*

Broadwell, M. (1969). *Teaching for learning (XVI)*. The Gospel Guardian.

Brown, A. N., Gilbert, B. J., Bruno, A. F., & Cooper, G. M. (2012). Validated competency framework for delivery of pharmacy services in pacific-Island countries. *Journal of Pharmacy Practice and Research*. doi:10.1002/j.2055-2335.2012.tb00186.x

Brunisholz, K. D., Olson, J., Anderson, J. W., Hays, E., Tilbury, P. M., Winter, B., ... Parkin, G. (2018). "Pharming out" support: A promising approach to integrating clinical pharmacists into established primary care medical home practices. *The Journal of International Medical Research*. Advance online publication. doi:10.1177/0300060517710885 PMID:28789606

Bruno-Tomé, A. (2018). *Teaching methodologies: the experience from Monash University*. Lisboa, Portugal: Academic Press.

Building a National Framework for the Establishment of Regulatory Science for Drug Development. (2011). In *Building a National Framework for the Establishment of Regulatory Science for Drug Development*. doi:10.17226/12968

Butterworth, J., Sansom, A., Sims, L., Healey, M., Kingsland, E., & Campbell, J. (2017). Pharmacists' perceptions of their emerging general practice roles in UK primary care: A qualitative interview study. *The British Journal of General Practice*. Advance online publication. doi:10.3399/bjgp17X691733 PMID:28673959

Cabral, A., Moura-Ramos, M., Castel-Branco, M., Caramona, M., Fernandez-Llimós, F., & Figueiredo, I. V. (2017). Influence of the mode of administration on the results of medication adherence questionnaires. *Journal of Evaluation in Clinical Practice*, *23*(6), 1–6. doi:10.1111/jep.12773 PMID:28714551

Cabral, M. D. J., Mamzer, M.-F., Hervé, C., Beecher Martins, C., & Charon, R. (2017). Narrative Medicine: What Discourse adds to Listening. *Anglo Saxonica*, *3*(13), 159–180.

Callréus, T., & Schneider, C. K. (2013). The emergence of regulatory science in pharmaceutical medicine. Pharmaceutical Medicine. doi:10.100740290-013-0039-x

Campbell, J., Dussault, G., Buchan, J., Pozo-Martin, F., Guerra Arias, M., Leone, C., . . . Cometto, G. A. (2013). *A universal truth: No health without a workforce*. Forum Report Third Global Forum on Human Resources for Health Global Health Workforce Alliance and World Health Organization.

Cantillon, P., & Sargeant, J. (2008). Giving feedback in clinical settings. *BMJ (Clinical Research Ed.)*, *337*(7681), 1292–1294. doi:10.1136/bmj.a1961 PMID:19001006

Carvalho, P. F., & Goldstone, R. L. (2015). The benefits of interleaved and blocked study: Different tasks benefit from different schedules of study. *Psychonomic Bulletin & Review*, *22*(1), 281–288. doi:10.375813423-014-0676-4 PMID:24984923

Casal, T. (2014). From Person to Patient: From Patient to Person? In P. Bray & T. Casal (Eds.), *Beyond Diagnosis: Relating the Person to the Patient - The Patient to the Person* (pp. 83–110). Inter-Disciplinary Press.

Case, E. (2005). Getting a Grip. *Ars Medici*, *2*(1), 76–79.

CEIC. (2016). *Ensaios Clínicos - Fluxograma de processo*. https://www.rnec.pt/submissao-nacional

CESIF. (2020). *Professional Expert Course Records and Regulatory Affairs*. https://www.healthcarestudies.com/Course-Professional-Expert-Drug-Registration-And-Regulatory-Affairs/Spain/CESIF/

Chapman, D. (2009). Advanced search features of PubMed. *Journal of the Canadian Academy of Child and Adolescent Psychiatry*, *18*(1), 58–59. PMID:19270851

Charon, R. (2001). Narrative Medicine: Form, Function, and Ethics. *Annals of Internal Medicine*, *134*(1), 83–87. doi:10.7326/0003-4819-134-1-200101020-00024 PMID:11187429

Charon, R. (2006). *Narrative Medicine: Honoring the Stories of Illness*. Oxford University Press, Inc., doi:10.7326/0003-4819-146-2-200701160-00021

Charon, R., Dasgupta, S., Hermann, N., Irvine, C., Marcus, E., Colón, E. R., ... Spiegel, M. (2017). *The principles and practice of narrative medicine. The Principles and Practice of Narrative Medicine*. Oxford University Press., doi:10.1080/10410236.2017.1403828

Charon, R., Hermann, N., & Devlin, M. J. (2016). Close Reading and Creative Writing in Clinical Education: Teaching Attention, Representation, and Affiliation. *Academic Medicine*, *91*(3), 345–350. doi:10.1097/ACM.0000000000000827 PMID:26200577

Chen, T. F. (2016). Pharmacist-Led Home Medicines Review and Residential Medication Management Review: The Australian Model. *Drugs & Aging*. Advance online publication. doi:10.100740266-016-0357-2 PMID:26961696

Chequeta, A., & Lewis, C. (2009). *How Providers Can Lower Costs and Improve Patient Care Using Evidence Based Medicine*. Oracle Corporation.

Cheung, M. W., & Vijayakumar, R. (2016). A Guide to Conducting a Meta-Analysis. *Neuropsychology Review*, *26*(2), 121–128. doi:10.100711065-016-9319-z PMID:27209412

Clauson, K. A., Marsh, W. A., Polen, H. H., Seamon, M. J., & Ortiz, B. I. (2007). Clinical decision support tools: Analysis of online drug information databases. *BMC Medical Informatics and Decision Making*, *7*(1), 7. doi:10.1186/1472-6947-7-7 PMID:17346336

Cole, T. R., Carlin, N. S., & Carson, R. A. (2015). Introducing Medical Humanities. *Medical Humanities: An Introduction*.

Cordina, M. (2019). Preparing the health workforce to enhance medication safety. *Research in Social & Administrative Pharmacy*, 813–814. PMID:30885570

Corrigan, T. (2012). *A Short Guide to Writing about Film* (8th ed.). Pearson.

Costa, F.A., Lee, V., Tous, S., Papastergiou, J., Neubeck, L., Freedman, B., & Antoniou, S. (2019). Awareness campaigns of Atrial Fibrillation as an opportunity for early detection by pharmacists- an international cross-sectional study. *Journal of Thrombosis and Thrombolysis*. . doi:10.100711239-019-02000-x

Costa, F., Scullin, C., Al-Anni, G., Hawwa, A., McElnay, J., Hersberger, K., & Westerlund, T. (2017). Provision of pharmaceutical care by community pharmacists across Europe: Is it developing and spreading? *Journal of Evaluation in Clinical Practice*, *23*(6), 1336–1347.

Crawford, N. D., Dean, T., Rivera, A. V., Guffey, T., Amesty, S., Rudolph, A., ... Fuller, C. M. (2016). Pharmacy intervention to improve HIV testing uptake using a comprehensive health screening approach. *Public Health Reports*. Advance online publication. doi:10.1177/00333549161310S116 PMID:26862239

Cummings, M. (1967). The role of the National Library of Medicine in the national biomedical library network. *Annals of the New York Academy of Sciences*, *142*(2), 503–512. doi:10.1111/j.1749-6632.1967.tb14365.x PMID:5230953

Damásio, A. (2011). *O erro de Descartes. Emoção, razão e cérebro humano*. Temas e Debates – Círculo de Leitores.

Davies, K., & Harrison, J. (2007). The information-seeking behaviour of doctors: A review of the evidence. *Health Information and Libraries Journal*, *24*(2), 78–94. doi:10.1111/j.1471-1842.2007.00713.x PMID:17584211

Davis, S., & Kruck, L. (1994). Drug information training and experience at U.S. schools of pharmacy. *American Journal of Pharmaceutical Education*, *58*(2).

de Sousa, I. C., de Lima David, J. P., & Noblat Lde, A. (2013). A drug information center module to train pharmacy students in evidence-based practice. *American Journal of Pharmaceutical Education*, *77*(4), 80. doi:10.5688/ajpe77480 PMID:23716748

Dee, C. (2007). The development of the Medical Literature Analysis and Retrieval System (MEDLARS). *Journal of the Medical Library Association: JMLA*, *95*(4), 416–425. doi:10.3163/1536-5050.95.4.416 PMID:17971889

Delwiche, F. A. (2008). Searching MEDLINE via PubMed. *Clinical Laboratory Science*, *21*(1), 35–41. PMID:18335860

Dewey, J. (1969). *The child and the curriculum and The school and Society joint edition*. University of Chicago Press, Phoenix Books.

Diário da República - Normas para atribuição do título de especialista em assuntos regulamentares. (2018) (testimony of Assembleia da República).

Dickinson, R., Raynor, D. K., Knapp, P., & MacDonald, J. (2017). How much information about the benefits of medicines is included in patient leaflets in the European Union? - A survey. *International Journal of Pharmacy Practice*, *25*(2), 147–158. doi:10.1111/ijpp.12285 PMID:27405658

dos Farmacêuticos, O. (2014). *Model for the Attribution of Pharmaceutical Competences and Specialties*. Obtido em 16 de 2 de 2019, de www.ordemfarmaceuticos.pt

dos Farmacêuticos, O. (2018). *Farmacêuticos em números*. Obtido em 23 de 11 de 2019, de https://www.ordemfarmaceuticos.pt/pt/numeros/

dos Farmacêuticos, O. (2018). *Ordem dos Farmacêuticos*. Obtido em 8 de 11 de 2019, de Regulamento interno de qualificação.: https://www.ordemfarmaceuticos.pt/fotos/documentos/regulamento_interno_de_qualificacao_versao_final_10071147805c1a3a94b2e41.pdf

dos Farmacêuticos, O. (2019). *Regulation for the Attribution of Pharmaceutical Competences*. Obtido de www.ordemfarmaceuticos.pt

dos Farmacêuticos, O., & Nacional, D. (2018). Reconhecimento de Formação de Farmacêuticos. Administração de vacinas e medicamentos injectáveis em farmácia comunitária.

Dos, L., Lima, S., & Cosme, A. (2017). *A metodologia de ensino-aprendizagem-avaliação através da resolução de problemas: O recorte de uma tese em desenvolvimento.* https://repositorio-aberto.up.pt/bitstream/10216/119397/2/322923.pdf

Drago, D., Shire, S., & Ekmekci, O. (2016). Improving Regulatory Education: Can We Reconcile Employers' Expectations With Academic Offerings? *Therapeutic Innovation & Regulatory Science, 50*(3), 330–336. Advance online publication. doi:10.1177/2168479015620440 PMID:30227069

Drews, J. (2000). Drug discovery: A historical perspective. *Science, 287*(5460), 1960–1964. doi:10.1126cience.287.5460.1960 PMID:10720314

Dreyfus, S. E. (2004). The five-stage model of adult skill acquisition. *Bulletin of Science, Technology & Society, 24*(3), 177–181. Advance online publication. doi:10.1177/0270467604264992

Duarte, M., Beecher Martins, C., & Pereira, P. (2019). *Application of Medical Humanities in Nursing Education - - The Design of Two Studies. 40th APEAA.*

EAFP. (2018). *Four Pillars for Relevant Pharmacy Education.* Position paper of the European Association of Faculties of Pharmacy 2018 Annual Conference, Parma, Italy.

Earl, G. L. (2009). Using cooperative learning for a drug information assignment. *American Journal of Pharmaceutical Education, 73*(7), 132. doi:10.5688/aj7307132 PMID:19960089

Eisenberg, M. (2008). Information Literacy: Essential Skills for the Information Age. *DESIDOC Journal of Library and Information Technology, 28*(2), 39–47. doi:10.14429/djlit.28.2.166

ESCP. (1988). *Clinical Pharmacy Education and Training for Pharmacists in the European Economic Community.* European Society of Clinical Pharmacy.

ESCP. (1993). *The future of Clinical Pharmacy in Europe: A strategy for the Society* (J. Bonal, M. Burden, & J. P. Delporte, Eds.). European Society of Clinical Pharmacy.

European Commission. (2013). *Diretiva 2013/55/UE do Parlamento Europeu e do Conselho, de 20 de novembro de 2013, que altera a Diretiva 2005/36/CE relativa ao reconhecimento das qualificações profissionais e o Regulamento (UE) n.o 1024/2012 relativo à cooperação administrativa através.* Jornal Oficial Da União Europeia.

European Commission. (2020). *EU R&D Scoreboard.* doi:10.2760/59430

European Medicines Agency. (2020a). *Advancing regulatory science in the EU – new strategy adopted.* Author.

European Medicines Agency. (2020b). *Human regulatory.* Clinical Trial Regulation.

European Medicines Agency. (n.d.). *Clinical Trials.* Author.

European Parliament. (2013). Directive 2013/55/EU of the European Parliament and of the council of 20 November 2013 amending Directive 2005/36/EC on the recognition of professional qualifications and Regulation. *Official Journal of the European Union*, (354), 132–170. Retrieved from https://eur-lex.europa.eu/LexUriServ/LexUriServ.do?uri=OJ:L:2013:354:0132:0170:en:PDF

European Pharmaceutical Students' Association. (n.d.). *Methodology Booklet*. Author.

European Pharmacy Students Association. (2018). *Methodology Booklet*. European Commission.

Evans, D. (2003). Hierarchy of evidence: A framework for ranking evidence evaluating healthcare interventions. *Journal of Clinical Nursing*, *12*(1), 77–84. doi:10.1046/j.1365-2702.2003.00662.x PMID:12519253

Eysenbach, G., Powell, J., Kuss, O., & Sa, E. R. (2002). Empirical studies assessing the quality of health information for consumers on the world wide web: A systematic review. *Journal of the American Medical Association*, *287*(20), 2691–2700. doi:10.1001/jama.287.20.2691 PMID:12020305

Farland, M. Z., Sicat, B. L., Franks, A. S., Pater, K. S., Medina, M. S., & Persky, A. M. (2013). Best Practices for Implementing Team-Based Learning in Pharmacy Education. *American Journal of Pharmaceutical Education*, *77*(8), 177. Advance online publication. doi:10.5688/ajpe778177 PMID:24159218

Fatmi, M., Hartling, L., Hillier, T., Campbell, S., & Oswald, A. E. (2013). The effectiveness of team-based learning on learning outcomes in health professions education: BEME Guide No. 30. *Medical Teacher*, *35*(12), e1608–e1624. doi:10.3109/0142159X.2013.849802 PMID:24245519

Federação Internacional Farmacêutica (FIP). (2017). *Transformar a formação e educação em farmácia e ciências farmacêuticas no contexto da força laboral farmacêutica*. Obtido em 18 de 2 de 2019, de https://fip.org/files/fip/PharmacyEducation/FIPEd_Nanjing_Report_2017_PT.pdf

Fernandez, R. S., Tran, D. T., Ramjan, L., Ho, C., & Gill, B. (2014). Comparison of four teaching methods on Evidence-based Practice skills of postgraduate nursing students. *Nurse Education Today*, *34*(1), 61–66. doi:10.1016/j.nedt.2012.10.005 PMID:23107585

Figueiredo, I. V., Castel-Branco, M., Fernandez-Llimós, F., & Caramona, M. (2018). Teaching topics in pharmaceutical care as a way to develop useful and practical research in community pharmacy. *Pharmacy Education: Towards Pharmaceutical Sciences*. Annual Conference of European Association of Faculties of Pharmacy. Parma, Italy.

FIP. (2008). *FIP's Vision, Mission and Strategic Plan*. Retrieved from https://www.fip.org/files/fip/strategic plan no annexes.pdf

FIP. (2014). *Access to medicines and pharmacists today, better outcomes tomorrow*. 74th World Congress of Pharmacy and Pharmaceutical Sciences. Bangkok, Thailand.

FIP. (2016a). *Global Vision for Education and Workforce Presented at the global conference on pharmacy and Pharmaceutical sciences education Nanjing Declaration Global Vision for a Global Pharmaceutical Workforce by Advancing Practice and Science through Transformative*. Retrieved from https://www.fip.org/files/fip/PharmacyEducation/2016_report/2016-11-Education-workforce-global-vision.pdf

FIP. (2016b). *Pharmaceutical Workforce Development Goals*. Retrieved from https://www.fip.org/files/content/priority-areas/workforce/wdgs-online-version.pdf

FIP. (2017). *Nanjing Statements.* Obtido em 06 de 12 de 2019, de https://www.fip.org/files/content/priorityareas/

FIP. (2017). *Nanjing Statements*. Retrieved from https://www.fip.org/files/content/priority-areas/workforce/nanjing-statements.pdf

FIP. (2019). *The FIP Workforce Transformation Programme (WTP)*. Retrieved from https://www.fip.org/files/fip/PharmacyEducation/2019/FIP-WTP-program-web.pdf

Fischer, J. M. (1980). Modification of the systematic approach to answering drug information requests. *American Journal of Hospital Pharmacy*, *37*(4), 470–476, 472, 476. doi:10.1093/ajhp/37.4.470 PMID:7377208

Flavell, J. H. (1979). Metacognition and Cognitive Monitoring: A New Area of Cognitive—Developmental Inquiry. *The American Psychologist*, *34*(10), 906–911. doi:10.1037/0003-066X.34.10.906

Food and Drug Administration. (2011). *Moving Regulatory Science into the 21st Century*. Advancing Regulatory Science at FDA.

Food and Drug Administration. (2018). *Step 3: Clinical Research | FDA*. https://www.fda.gov/patients/drug-development-process/step-3-clinical-research

Food and Drug Administration. (2020). *FDA Regulations Relating to Good Clinical Practice and Clinical Trials. Regulations: Good Clinical Practice and Clinical Trials*. Author.

Frank, J. R., Mungroo, R., Ahmad, Y., Wang, M., De Rossi, S., & Horsley, T. (2010). Toward a definition of competency-based education in medicine: A systematic review of published definitions. *Medical Teacher*, *32*(8), 631–637. Advance online publication. doi:10.3109/0142159X.2010.500898 PMID:20662573

Freeman, S., Eddy, S. L., McDonough, M., Smith, M. K., Okoroafor, N., Jordt, H., & Wenderoth, M. P. (2014). Active learning increases student performance in science, engineering, and mathematics. *Proceedings of the National Academy of Sciences of the United States of America*. 10.1073/pnas.1319030111

Ghaibi, S., Ipema, H., & Gabay, M. (2015). ASHP Guidelines on the Pharmacist's Role in Providing Drug Information. *American Journal of Health-System Pharmacy*, *72*(7), 573–577. doi:10.2146p150002 PMID:25788512

Girvin, B. W. D. (2018). Clinical skills training for pharmacists in general practice. *The Prescriber*, 19–25.

Gonzalez-Gonzalez, A. I., Dawes, M., Sanchez-Mateos, J., Riesgo-Fuertes, R., Escortell-Mayor, E., Sanz-Cuesta, T., & Hernandez-Fernandez, T. (2007). Information needs and information-seeking behavior of primary care physicians. *Annals of Family Medicine*, *5*(4), 345–352. doi:10.1370/afm.681 PMID:17664501

Gonzalez, J., Bryant, S., Hogan, M., Bai, S., Fierro, L., & Hermes-DeSantis, E. R. (2019). Comparison of Postdoctoral Pharmacy Training Programs: Drug Information Residencies and Medical Information Fellowships. *Therapeutic Innovation & Regulatory Science*, *53*(4), 446–454. doi:10.1177/2168479018793375 PMID:30176737

Goodman-snitkoff, G., & Snitkoff, L. S. (2006). Use of Enriched Case Studies to Enhance Empathy in Pharmacy Students. *Journal of Pharmacy Teaching*, *13*(2), 5–16. doi:10.1300/J060v13n02_02

Greca, I. M., & Moreira, M. A. (2000). Mental models, conceptual models and modeling. *International Journal of Science Education*, *22*(1), 1–11. doi:10.1080/095006900289976

Gubbins, P. O. M. S. (2014). Innovation in clinical pharmacy practice and opportunities for academic—practice partnership. *Pharmacotherapy, 34*(5), 45-54. http://bte.gep.msess.gov.pt/separatas/sep33_2019.pdf

Guskey, T.R. (n.d.). *Evaluating professional development.* University of Kentucky.

Guyatt, G. H., Oxman, A. D., Kunz, R., Falck-Ytter, Y., Vist, G. E., Liberati, A., ... Group, G. W. (2008). Going from evidence to recommendations. *BMJ (Clinical Research Ed.)*, *336*(7652), 1049–1051. doi:10.1136/bmj.39493.646875.AE PMID:18467413

Guyatt, G. H., Oxman, A. D., Kunz, R., Vist, G. E., Falck-Ytter, Y., & Schünemann, H. J. (2008). GRADE: What is "quality of evidence" and why is it important to clinicians? *BMJ (Clinical Research Ed.)*, *336*(7651), 995–998. doi:10.1136/bmj.39490.551019.BE PMID:18456631

Guyatt, G. H., Oxman, A. D., Vist, G. E., Kunz, R., Falck-Ytter, Y., Alonso-Coello, P., ... Group, G. W. (2008). GRADE: An emerging consensus on rating quality of evidence and strength of recommendations. *BMJ (Clinical Research Ed.)*, *336*(7650), 924–926. doi:10.1136/bmj.39489.470347.AD PMID:18436948

Haghparast, N., Sedghizadeh, P. P., Shuler, C. F., Ferati, D., & Christersson, C. (2007). Evaluation of student and faculty perceptions of the PBL curriculum at two dental schools from a student perspective: A cross-sectional survey. *European Journal of Dental Education*, *11*(1), 14–22. Advance online publication. doi:10.1111/j.1600-0579.2007.00423.x PMID:17227391

Haidet, P., Levine, R. E., Parmelee, D. X., Crow, S., Kennedy, F., Kelly, P. A., Perkowski, L., Michaelsen, L., & Richards, B. F. (2012). Perspective: Guidelines for reporting team-based learning activities in the medical and health sciences education literature. Academic Medicine. doi:10.1097/ACM.0b013e318244759e

Hamburg, M. A. (2011). Advancing Regulatory Science. Science. doi:10.1126cience.1204432

Hasan, S. (2011). Teaching ethics to pharmacy students using a team-based learning approach. *Pharmacy Education, 11*(1), 99–106.

Hatala, R., & Guyatt, G. (2002). Evaluating the teaching of evidence-based medicine. *Journal of the American Medical Association, 288*(9), 1110–1112. doi:10.1001/jama.288.9.1110 PMID:12204080

Hazen, A. C. M., de Bont, A. A., Boelman, L., Zwart, D. L. M., de Gier, J. J., de Wit, N. J., & Bouvy, M. L. (2018). The degree of integration of non-dispensing pharmacists in primary care practice and the impact on health outcomes: A systematic review. *Research in Social & Administrative Pharmacy*. Advance online publication. doi:10.1016/j.sapharm.2017.04.014 PMID:28506574

Hepler, C. D., & Strand, L. M. (1990). Opportunities and responsibilities in pharmaceutical care. *American Journal of Hospital Pharmacy*. Advance online publication. doi:10.1093/ajhp/47.3.533 PMID:2316538

Herdeiro, M. T., Teixeira Rodrigues, A., Ferreira, M., da Cruz e Silva, O. A. B., & Fardilha, M. (2014). Multi-method active learning approach: Improving the educational experience in pharmaceutical drug development. *Indian Journal of Pharmaceutical Education and Research*. doi:10.5530/ijper.48.3.4

Herner, M. (2019). Perfect Top of the Evidence Hierarchy Pyramid, Maybe Not So Perfect: Lessons learned by a novice researcher engaging in a meta-analysis project. *BMJ Evidence-Based Medicine, 24*(4), 130–132. doi:10.1136/bmjebm-2018-111141 PMID:30842066

Hersh, W. R., Gorman, P. N., Biagioli, F. E., Mohan, V., Gold, J. A., & Mejicano, G. C. (2014). Beyond information retrieval and electronic health record use: Competencies in clinical informatics for medical education. *Advances in Medical Education and Practice, 5*, 205–212. doi:10.2147/AMEP.S63903 PMID:25057246

Higgins, J. P. T., & Green, S. (Eds.). (2011). *Cochrane Handbook for Systematic Reviews of Interventions Version 5.1.0* [updated March 2011]. The Cochrane Collaboration. Available from www.handbook.cochrane.org

Higgins, J. P., Altman, D. G., Gotzsche, P. C., Juni, P., Moher, D., Oxman, A. D., ... Cochrane Statistical Methods, G. (2011). The Cochrane Collaboration's tool for assessing risk of bias in randomised trials. *BMJ (Clinical Research Ed.), 343*(oct18 2), d5928. doi:10.1136/bmj.d5928 PMID:22008217

Hines, P. A., Guy, R. H., Humphreys, A. J., & Papaluca-Amati, M. (2019). The European Medicines Agency's goals for regulatory science to 2025. Nature Reviews Drug Discovery. doi:10.1038/d41573-019-00071-2

Hines, P. A., Gonzalez-Quevedo, R., Lambert, A. I. O. M., Janssens, R., Freischem, B., Torren Edo, J., Claassen, I. J. T. M., & Humphreys, A. J. (2020). Regulatory Science to 2025: An Analysis of Stakeholder Responses to the European Medicines Agency's Strategy. *Frontiers in Medicine, 7*, 508. Advance online publication. doi:10.3389/fmed.2020.00508 PMID:33072771

Hines, P. A., Guy, R. H., Brand, A., Humphreys, A. J., & Papaluca-Amati, M. (2019). Regulatory Science and Innovation Programme for Europe (ReScIPE): A proposed model. *Journal of Clinical Pharmacology*. PMID:31426120

Hirvonen, J., Salminen, O., Vuorensola, K., Katajavuori, N., Huhtala, H., & Atkinson, J. (2019). Pharmacy Practice and Education in Finland. *Pharmacy (Basel, Switzerland)*, *7*(1), 21. Advance online publication. doi:10.3390/pharmacy7010021 PMID:30813453

Hojat, M., Vergare, M. J., Maxwell, K., Brainard, G., Herrine, S. K., Isenberg, G. A., Veloski, J., & Gonnella, J. S. (2009). The devil is in the third year: A longitudinal study of erosion of empathy in medical school. *Academic Medicine*, *84*(9), 1182–1191. doi:10.1097/ACM.0b013e3181b17e55 PMID:19707055

Hooker, C. (2008). The medical humanities: A brief introduction. *Australian Family Physician*, *37*(5), 369–370. PMID:18464968

Hooker, C. (2014). Ethics and the arts in the medical humanities. In P. Macneill (Ed.), *Ethics and the Arts* (pp. 213–224). Springer., doi:10.1007/978-94-017-8816-8_19

Horntvedt, M. T., Nordsteien, A., Fermann, T., & Severinsson, E. (2018). Strategies for teaching evidence-based practice in nursing education: A thematic literature review. *BMC Medical Education*, *18*(1), 172. doi:10.118612909-018-1278-z PMID:30055612

Huedo-Medina, T. B., Sanchez-Meca, J., Marin-Martinez, F., & Botella, J. (2006). Assessing heterogeneity in meta-analysis: Q statistic or I2 index? *Psychological Methods*, *11*(2), 193–206. doi:10.1037/1082-989X.11.2.193 PMID:16784338

Hung, H. Y., Wang, Y. W., Feng, J. Y., Wang, C. J., Lin, E. C., & Chang, Y. J. (2019). Evidence-Based Practice Curriculum Development for Undergraduate Nursing Students: The Preliminary Results of an Action Research Study in Taiwan. *The Journal of Nursing Research*, *27*(4), e30. doi:10.1097/jnr.0000000000000298 PMID:30461524

Hurst, J. (2000). Challenges for health in member countries of the organisation for economic co-operation and development. *Bulletin of the World Health Organization*. doi:10.1590/S0042-96862000000600007

Hurwitz, B. (2015). Medical Humanities: Origins, Orientations and Contributions. *Anglo Saxonica III*, *10*, 10–31.

Hurwitz, B., & Dakin, P. (2009). Welcome developments in UK medical humanities. *Journal of the Royal Society of Medicine*, *102*(3), 84–85. doi:10.1258/jrsm.2009.080383 PMID:19297643

Ilcewicz, H. N., Poirier, T. I., & Pailden, J. (2018). Use of mixed-methods approach to assess the impact of a pre- professional health humanities honors course on developing interpersonal skills. *Currents in Pharmacy Teaching & Learning*, *10*(11), 1456–1465. doi:10.1016/j.cptl.2018.08.010 PMID:30514535

Imfeld-Isenegger, T. L. S. I. (2019). Pharmacist-led medication review procedures: a survey across Europe. Research in Social and Administrative Pharmacy. doi:10.1016/j.sapharm.2019.11.002

Imfeld-Isenegger, T. L., Soares, I. B., & Hersberger, K. E. (2019). Pharmacist-led medication review procedures: a survey across Europe. Research in Social and Administrative Pharmacy. doi:10.1016/j.saph

INFARMED. (2017). *Estatísticas de avaliação de ensaios clínicos pelo Infarmed*. https://www.infarmed.pt/web/infarmed/entidades/medicamentos-uso-humano/ensaios-clinicos/estatisticas

Institute of Medicine (US) Forum on Drug Discovery Development and Translation. (2011). *Building a National Framework for the Establishment of Regulatory Science for Drug Development: Workshop Summary*. Author.

International Conference on Harmonisation of Technical Requirements for Registration of Pharmaceuticals for Human Use. (1997). *General Considerations for Clinical Trials E8*. Author.

International Pharmaceutical Federation (FIP). (2017a). *Pharmacy as a Gateway to care: helping people towards better health*. Author.

International Pharmaceutical Federation (FIP). (2017b). *Reducing harm associated with drugs of abuse: the role of pharmacists*. Author.

International Pharmaceutical Federation (FIP). (2018). *Pharmacists supporting women and the responsible use of medicines*. Author.

International Pharmaceutical Federation. (2012). *FIP Education Initiatives*. A Global Competency Framework for Services Provided by Pharmacy Workforce. Version 1.

International Pharmaceutical Federation. (2015). *Global trends shaping pharmacy - Regulatory Frameworks, Distribution of Medicines and Professional Services, 2013-2015*. Author.

International Pharmaceutical Federation. (2017). *Pharmacy at a Glance 2015-2017*. Author.

International Pharmaceutical Federation. (2019). *Beating non-communicable diseases in the community: The contribution of pharmacists*. Author.

IntHout, J., Ioannidis, J. P. A., Rovers, M. M., & Goeman, J. J. (2016). Plea for routinely presenting prediction intervals in meta-analysis. *BMJ Open*, *6*(7), e010247. doi:10.1136/bmjopen-2015-010247 PMID:27406637

Ioannidis, J. P. A. (2016). Why Most Clinical Research Is Not Useful. *PLoS Medicine*, *13*(6), e1002049. Advance online publication. doi:10.1371/journal.pmed.1002049 PMID:27328301

Iwanowicz, S. L., Marciniak, M. W., & Zeolla, M. M. (2006). Obtaining and providing health information in the community pharmacy setting. *American Journal of Pharmaceutical Education*, *70*(3), 57. doi:10.5688/aj700357 PMID:17136178

Jansen, W. (2019). *Problem-based Learning at Maastricht University. Academic Press.*

Jiménez-Saiz, R., & Rosace, D. (2019). Is hybrid-PBL advancing teaching in biomedicine? A systematic review. BMC Medical Education. doi:10.118612909-019-1673-0

Kasworm, C. (2011). New perspectives on post-formal cognitive development and self-directed learning. *International Journal of Self-Directed Learning*, *8*(1).

Katoue, M. G., & Schwinghammer, T. L. (2020). Competency-based education in pharmacy: A review of its development, applications, and challenges. *Journal of Evaluation in Clinical Practice*, *26*(4), 1–10. doi:10.1111/jep.13362 PMID:32069376

Kearney, R. (2004). *On Stories: Thinking in Action*. Routledge.

Kennedy, D. R. (2019). Redesigning a pharmacology course to promote active learning. *American Journal of Pharmaceutical Education*, *83*(5), 6782. Advance online publication. doi:10.5688/ajpe6782 PMID:31333258

Khan, K. S., & Coomarasamy, A. (2006). A hierarchy of effective teaching and learning to acquire competence in evidenced-based medicine. *BMC Medical Education*, *6*(1), 59. doi:10.1186/1472-6920-6-59 PMID:17173690

Kibble, J. D., Bellew, C., Asmar, A., & Barkley, L. (2016). Team-based learning in large enrollment classes. *Advances in Physiology Education*, *40*(4), 435–442. doi:10.1152/advan.00095.2016 PMID:27697956

Kier, K., & Goldwire, M. (2018). Drug Information Resources and Literature Retrieval (7th ed.). ACCP's Pharmacotherapy Self-Assessment Program.

Kirkdale, C. L., Nebout, G., Megerlin, F., & Thornley, T. (2017). Benefits of pharmacist-led flu vaccination services in community pharmacy. *Annales Pharmaceutiques Francaises*. Advance online publication. doi:10.1016/j.pharma.2016.08.005 PMID:27717412

Koster, A., Schalekamp, T., & Meijerman, I. (2017). Implementation of competency based pharmacy education (CBPE). *Pharmacy (Basel, Switzerland)*, *5*(1), 10. doi:10.3390/pharmacy5010010 PMID:28970422

Kruger, J., & Dunning, D. (1999). Unskilled and unaware of it: How difficulties in recognizing one's own incompetence lead to inflated self-assessments. *Journal of Personality and Social Psychology*, *77*(6), 1121–1134. doi:10.1037/0022-3514.77.6.1121 PMID:10626367

Krug, R. de R., Vieira, M. S. M., & Maciel, M. V. de A. e, Erdmann, T. R., Vieira, F. C. de F., Koch, M. C., & Grosseman, S. (2016). O "Bê-Á-Bá" da Aprendizagem Baseada em Equipe. *Revista Brasileira de Educação Médica*, *40*(4), 602–610. doi:10.1590/1981-52712015v40n4e00452015

Kuster, M., De Tonnac, A., & Papa, S. (2019). How to write a case-report? *Revue Medicale Suisse*, *15*(664), 1699–1702. PMID:31553533

Kyriakoulis, K., Patelarou, A., Laliotis, A., Wan, A. C., Matalliotakis, M., Tsiou, C., & Patelarou, E. (2016). Educational strategies for teaching evidence-based practice to undergraduate health students: Systematic review. *Journal of Educational Evaluation for Health Professions*, *13*, 34. doi:10.3352/jeehp.2016.13.34 PMID:27649902

Kyu, H. H., Abate, D., Abate, K. H., Abay, S. M., Abbafati, C., Abbasi, N., ... Murray, C. J. L. (2018). Global, regional, and national disability-adjusted life-years (DALYs) for 359 diseases and injuries and healthy life expectancy (HALE) for 195 countries and territories, 1990-2017: A systematic analysis for the Global Burden of Disease Study 2017. *Lancet*. Advance online publication. doi:10.1016/S0140-6736(18)32335-3 PMID:30415748

Lang, B., Zhang, L., Lin, Y., Han, L., Zhang, C., & Liu, Y. (2019). Team-based learning pedagogy enhances the quality of Chinese pharmacy education: A systematic review and meta-analysis. *BMC Medical Education*, *19*(1), 286. doi:10.118612909-019-1724-6 PMID:31357986

Langdon, J., Botnaru, D. T., Wittenberg, M., Riggs, A. J., Mutchler, J., Syno, M., & Caciula, M. C. (2019). Examining the effects of different teaching strategies on metacognition and academic performance. *Advances in Physiology Education*, *43*(3), 414–422. doi:10.1152/advan.00013.2018 PMID:31408387

Larsen, C. M., Terkelsen, A. S., Carlsen, A. F., & Kristensen, H. K. (2019). Methods for teaching evidence-based practice: A scoping review. *BMC Medical Education*, *19*(1), 259. doi:10.118612909-019-1681-0 PMID:31296212

Law, M., Bader, L., Uzman, N., Williams, A., & Bates, I. (2019). *The FIP Nanjing Statements: Shaping global pharmacy and pharmaceutical sciences education. In Research in Social and Administrative Pharmacy*. Elsevier Inc., doi:10.1016/j.sapharm.2019.03.013

Lei n.º 21/2014, de 16 de abril, (2014) (testimony of INFARMED). https://www.infarmed.pt/documents/15786/1068535/036-B1_Lei_21_2014_1alt.pdf

Leppink, J., & van den Heuvel, A. (2015). The evolution of cognitive load theory and its application to medical education. *Perspectives on Medical Education*, *4*(3), 119–127. doi:10.100740037-015-0192-x PMID:26016429

Levine, R. E., Hsieh, P., Kelly, P. A., Carchedi, L., Gibson, J., Haidet, P., ... Thompson, B. (2019). The Facilitator Instrument for Team-Based Learning (FIT). *Teaching and Learning in Medicine*, *1334*. Advance online publication. doi:10.1080/10401334.2019.1646653 PMID:31389259

Lindberg, D. (2000). Internet access to the National Library of Medicine. Effective clinical practice. *ECP*, *3*(5), 256–260. PMID:11185333

Long, J. D., Gannaway, P., Ford, C., Doumit, R., Zeeni, N., Sukkarieh-Haraty, O., Milane, A., Byers, B., Harrison, L. N., Hatch, D., Brown, J., Proper, S., White, P., & Song, H. (2016). Effectiveness of a Technology-Based Intervention to Teach Evidence-Based Practice: The EBR Tool. *Worldviews on Evidence-Based Nursing*, *13*(1), 59–65. doi:10.1111/wvn.12132 PMID:26773417

Lorenzoni, L., Marino, A., Morgan, D., & James, C. (2019). *Health Spending Projections to 2030*. Academic Press.

Lumpkin, M. M., Eichler, H. G., Breckenridge, A., Hamburg, M. A., Lönngren, T., & Woods, K. (2012). Advancing the science of medicines regulation: The role of the 21st-century medicines regulator. Clinical Pharmacology and Therapeutics. doi:10.1038/clpt.2012.146

Lyn Corno, E. M. (2015). *Handbook of Educational Psychology*. Routledge. doi:10.4324/9781315688244

Malone, P., Kier, K., Stanovich, J. E., & Malone, M. J. (2014). *Drug Information: A Guide for Pharmacists* (5th ed.). McGraw-Hill Education.

Manasse, H. R., Brock, T., & Gal, D. (2009). *WHO UNESCO FIP Pharmacy Education Taskforce 4th Annual Global Pharmacy Education Consultation Report*? Retrieved from www.fip.org/education

Manasse, H. (1990). A philosophy of education in the next millennium. *Conference on Lifelong Learning in Pharmacy*, Copenhagen, Denmark.

Manasse, H. R. Jr. (2005). ASHP s 2015 initiative: A collective effort to improve pharmacy practice in hospitals and health-systems in the United States. *Farmacia Hospitalaria*, *29*(6), 349–350. doi:10.1016/S1130-6343(05)73693-X PMID:16433564

Martin, B. A., Porter, A. L., Shawl, L., & Motl Moroney, S. E. (2012). A model for partnering first-year student pharmacists with community-based older adults. *American Journal of Pharmaceutical Education*, *76*(5), 85. Advance online publication. doi:10.5688/ajpe76585 PMID:22761526

Martins, S., van Mil, J. W. F., & Costa, F. A. (2015). The Organizational Framework of Community Pharmacies in Europe. *International Journal of Clinical Pharmacy*, *37*(5), 896–905. doi:10.100711096-015-0140-1 PMID:26017399

Mary, S., Julie, J., & Jennifer, G. (2014). Teaching evidence based practice and research through blended learning to undergraduate midwifery students from a practice based perspective. *Nurse Education in Practice*, *14*(2), 220–224. doi:10.1016/j.nepr.2013.10.001 PMID:24189434

Mears, G. (2009). Avoid information overload. Now that you have data, What do you do with it? *JEMS: A Journal of Emergency Medical Services*, *34*(8), 12–15. PMID:19718851

Medical University of Vienna. (n.d.). *The MRA: European Master of Regulatory Affairs*. Retrieved October 1, 2020, from http://www.emtrain.eu/index.php/news/410-the-mra-european-master-of-regulatory-affairs

Mekonnen, A. B., McLachlan, A. J., & Brien, J. A. E. (2016). Effectiveness of pharmacist-led medication reconciliation programmes on clinical outcomes at hospital transitions: A systematic review and meta-analysis. *BMJ Open*. Advance online publication. doi:10.1136/bmjopen-2015-010003 PMID:26908524

Mennenga, H. (2012). Development and Psychometric Testing of the Team-Based Learning Student Assessment Instrument. *Nurse Educator*, *37*(4), 168–172. doi:10.1097/NNE.0b013e31825a87cc PMID:22688878

Merigo, J. M., & Nunez, A. (2016). Influential journals in health research: A bibliometric study. *Globalization and Health*, *12*(1), 46. doi:10.118612992-016-0186-4 PMID:27550071

Michaelsen, L. K. (2002). Getting started with team-based learning. In *Team-based learning: a transformative use of small groups* (pp. 27–51). Praeger Publisher.

Miranda, G. F., Vercellesi, L., & Bruno, F. (2004). Information sources in biomedical science and medical journalism: Methodological approaches and assessment. *Pharmacological Research*, *50*(3), 267–272. doi:10.1016/j.phrs.2003.12.021 PMID:15225669

Moghissi, A., Calderone, R., Auffret, J. P., Jaeger, L., Longstreth, J., McBride, D., Steen, T., Harrison, D., Garrison, D., & McDaniel, N. (2020). Regulatory Science Education: The Need for Generalization. *Journal of Regional Science*, *8*, 1–7.

Moher, D., Liberati, A., Tetzlaff, J., Altman, D. G., & Group, P. (2009). Preferred reporting items for systematic reviews and meta-analyses: The PRISMA statement. *BMJ (Clinical Research Ed.)*, *339*(jul21 1), b2535. doi:10.1136/bmj.b2535 PMID:19622551

Mona Mourshed, D. F. (2012). *Education to Employment: Designing a system that works*. McKinsey Center for Government.

Mononen, N., Jarvinen, R., Hameen-Anttila, K., Airaksinen, M., Bonhomme, C., Kleme, J., & Pohjanoksa-Mantyla, M. (2018). A national approach to medicines information research: A systematic review. *Research in Social & Administrative Pharmacy*, *14*(12), 1106–1124. Advance online publication. doi:10.1016/j.sapharm.2018.01.011 PMID:29483046

Montgomery, K. (2006). *How Doctors Think: Clinical Judgement and the Practice of Medicine*. OUP.

Morais, J. G., & Caramona, M. M. (2019). Creative Education: towards competences in a patient pharmacy education. *25th Annual conference of EAFP*. Closing session conference, Krakow, Poland.

MPharm in Pharmacy. (2019). Obtido de University of Strathclyde, Scotland: https://www.strath.ac.uk/courses/undergraduate/pharmacy/

Mueller, S. K., Sponsler, K. C., Kripalani, S., & Schnipper, J. L. (2012). Hospital-based medication reconciliation practices: A systematic review. *Archives of Internal Medicine*. Advance online publication. doi:10.1001/archinternmed.2012.2246 PMID:22733210

Mugo, P. M., Micheni, M., Shangala, J., Hussein, M. H., Graham, S. M., Rinke De Wit, T. F., & Sanders, E. J. (2017). Uptake and acceptability of oral HIV self-testing among community pharmacy clients in Kenya: A feasibility study. *PLoS One*. Advance online publication. doi:10.1371/journal.pone.0170868 PMID:28125699

Murad, M. H., Asi, N., Alsawas, M., & Alahdab, F. (2016). New evidence pyramid. *Evidence-Based Medicine*, *21*(4), 125–127. doi:10.1136/ebmed-2016-110401 PMID:27339128

Nachtigal, P., Šimůnek, T., & Atkinson, J. (2017). Pharmacy Practice and Education in the Czech Republic. *Pharmacy (Basel, Switzerland)*, *5*(4), 54. Advance online publication. doi:10.3390/pharmacy5040054 PMID:28991203

Naß, J., Banerjee, M., Efferth, T., & Wohlmann, A. (2016). Pharmaceutical care as narrative practice? Rethinking patient-centered care through a pharmacist's perspective. *International Journal of Clinical Pharmacy*, *38*(6), 1346–1349. doi:10.100711096-016-0391-5 PMID:27766501

Nathan, J. P. (2013). Drug information—the systematic approach: Continuing education article. *Journal of Pharmacy Practice*, *26*(2), 78–84. doi:10.1177/0897190012474229 PMID:23519502

National Library of Medicine. (2019). *MeSH (Medical Subject Headings)*. https://www.ncbi.nlm.nih.gov/mesh

Nation, L. M., Tweddell, S., & Rutter, P. (2016). The applicability of a validated team-based learning student assessment instrument to assess United Kingdom pharmacy students' attitude toward team-based learning. *Journal of Educational Evaluation for Health Professions*, *13*, 30. doi:10.3352/jeehp.2016.13.30 PMID:27568493

Nkansah, N., Mostovetsky, O., Yu, C., Chheng, T., Beney, J., Bond, C. M., & Bero, L. (2010). Effect of outpatient pharmacists' non-dispensing roles on patient outcomes and prescribing patterns. *Cochrane Database of Systematic Reviews*, (7), CD000336. doi:10.1002/14651858.CD000336.pub2 PMID:20614422

Northwest Center for Public Health Practice at the University of Washington School of Public Health. (2014). *Effective Adult Learning. A toolkit for teaching adults*. Robert Wood Johnson Foundation.

Novak, C. J., Hastanan, S., Moradi, M., & Terry, D. F. (2012). Reducing unnecessary hospital readmissions: The pharmacist's role in care transitions. *The Consultant Pharmacist*. Advance online publication. doi:10.4140/TCP.n.2012.174 PMID:22421517

Nunes-Da-Cunha, I., Arguello, B., Martinez, F. M., & Fernandez-Llimos, F. (2016). A comparison of patient-centered care in pharmacy curricula in the United States and Europe. *American Journal of Pharmaceutical Education*, *80*(5), 83. Advance online publication. doi:10.5688/ajpe80583 PMID:27402986

Oberauer, K., & Lewandowsky, S. (2008). Forgetting in immediate serial recall: Decay, temporal distinctiveness, or interference? *Psychological Review*, *115*(3), 544–576. doi:10.1037/0033-295X.115.3.544 PMID:18729591

OECD. (2017). *Health at a Glance: Pharmaceutical Sector.* OECD.

Organization, W. H. (2011). *Joint FIP/WHO Guidelines on Good Pharmacy Practice: Standards for quality of pharmacy services. Geneva 2011*. Report.

Papastergiou, J., Folkins, C., Li, W., & Zervas, J. (2014). Community pharmacist–administered influenza immunization improves patient access to vaccination. *Canadian Pharmacists Journal*. Advance online publication. doi:10.1177/1715163514552557 PMID:25364353

Parmelee, D., Michaelsen, L. K., Cook, S., & Hudes, P. D. (2012). Team-based learning: A practical guide: AMEE Guide No. 65. *Medical Teacher*, *34*(5), 275–288. doi:10.3109/0142159X.2012.651179 PMID:22471941

Patelarou, A. E., Kyriakoulis, K. G., Stamou, A. A., Laliotis, A., Sifaki-Pistolla, D., Matalliotakis, M., Prokopakis, E., & Patelarou, E. (2017). Approaches to teach evidence-based practice among health professionals: An overview of the existing evidence. *Advances in Medical Education and Practice*, *8*, 455–464. doi:10.2147/AMEP.S134475 PMID:28740443

Pêgo, A., Pereira, A. da C., Figueiredo, A., Araújo, A., Severiano, A. I., Macedo, A., Anes, A. M., Silva, A. M., Moreira, A., Paróla, A., Duarte, A. P., Martins, A. P., Martins, A. S., Vaz, A. F., Lourenço, A., Gouveia, A. M., de Araújo, A. V. R., Torre, C., Ribeiro, C. F., . . . Maria, V. A. (2018). Farmacovigilância em Portugal: 25 anos. In *Farmacovigilância em Portugal: 25 anos*. http://app10.infarmed.pt/e_book_farmacovigilancia25/index.html

Pennycook, G., Ross, R. M., Koehler, D. J., & Fugelsang, J. A. (2017). Dunning-Kruger effects in reasoning: Theoretical implications of the failure to recognize incompetence. *Psychonomic Bulletin & Review*, *24*(6), 1774–1784. doi:10.375813423-017-1242-7 PMID:28224482

Petkova, V., & Atkinson, J. (2017). Pharmacy Practice and Education in Bulgaria. *Pharmacy (Basel, Switzerland)*, *5*(4), 35. Advance online publication. doi:10.3390/pharmacy5030035 PMID:28970446

Phillips, D. C., & Soltis, J. F. (2009). *Perspectives on Learning*. Teachers College Press, Columbia University.

Phillips, J. A., Gabay, M. P., Ficzere, C., & Ward, K. E. (2012). Curriculum and instructional methods for drug information, literature evaluation, and biostatistics: Survey of US pharmacy schools. *The Annals of Pharmacotherapy*, *46*(6), 793–801. doi:10.1345/aph.1Q813 PMID:22669797

Piaget, J. (1969). *Psychology of Intelligence*. Littlefield, Adams.

Pires, C., & Cavaco, A. (2019). Scoping Pharmacy Students' Learning Outcomes: Where Do We Stand? *Pharmacy (Basel, Switzerland)*, *7*(1), 23. Advance online publication. doi:10.3390/pharmacy7010023 PMID:30818854

Poirier, T. I., Stamper-Carr, C., & Newman, K. (2017). A course for developing interprofessional skills in pre-professional honor students using humanities and media. *Currents in Pharmacy Teaching & Learning*, *9*(5), 874–880. doi:10.1016/j.cptl.2017.05.004 PMID:29233318

Postma, T. C., & White, J. G. (2017). Students' perceptions of vertical and horizontal integration in a discipline-based dental school? *European Journal of Dental Education*, *21*(2), 101–107. doi:10.1111/eje.12186 PMID:26801357

Ramis, M. A., Chang, A., Conway, A., Lim, D., Munday, J., & Nissen, L. (2019). Theory-based strategies for teaching evidence-based practice to undergraduate health students: A systematic review. *BMC Medical Education*, *19*(1), 267. doi:10.118612909-019-1698-4 PMID:31319892

Rapport, F., Doel, M. A., Hutchings, H. A., Wright, S., Wainwright, P., John, D. N., & Jerzembek, G. S. (2010). Eleven themes of patient-centred professionalism in community pharmacy: Innovative approaches to consulting. *International Journal of Pharmacy Practice*, *18*(5), 260–268. doi:10.1111/j.2042-7174.2010.00056.x PMID:20840681

Rasi, G. (2017). *EU's innovative medical technology and EMA's measures*. Symposium, Presented at Summit of Heads of Medicines Regulatory Agencies (ICMRA)., and International Coalition of Medicines Regulatory Authorities.

Redwanski, J. (2012). Incorporating Team-Based Learning in a Drug Information Course Covering Tertiary Literature. *Currents in Pharmacy Teaching & Learning*, *4*(3), 202–206. doi:10.1016/j.cptl.2012.04.004

Reimschisel, T., Herring, A. L., Huang, J., & Minor, T. J. (2017). A systematic review of the published literature on team-based learning in health professions education. *Medical Teacher*, *39*(12), 1–11. doi:10.1080/0142159X.2017.1340636 PMID:28664760

Rosenberg, J. M., Koumis, T., Nathan, J. P., Cicero, L. A., & McGuire, H. (2004). Current status of pharmacist-operated drug information centers in the United States. *American Journal of Health-System Pharmacy*, *61*(19), 2023–2032. doi:10.1093/ajhp/61.19.2023 PMID:15509125

Rosenblatt, L. (2005). Case Study Monologue. *Ars Medici*, *2*(1), 34–44.

Rotellar, C., & Cain, J. (2016). Research, perspectives, and recommendations on implementing the flipped classroom. *American Journal of Pharmaceutical Education*, *80*(2), 34. Advance online publication. doi:10.5688/ajpe80234 PMID:27073287

Rouse, M. J. (2004). Continuing Professional Development in Pharmacy. *The Journal of Pharmacy Technology*, *20*(5), 303–306. doi:10.1177/875512250402000509

Sackett, D. L., Rosenberg, W. M., Gray, J. A., Haynes, R. B., & Richardson, W. S. (1996). Evidence based medicine: What it is and what it isn't. *BMJ (Clinical Research Ed.)*, *312*(7023), 71–72. doi:10.1136/bmj.312.7023.71 PMID:8555924

Sando, K. R., & Feng, X. (2018). Use of an Online Spaced-Education Game to Study Top 200 Drugs in a Skills Laboratory Course. *American Journal of Pharmaceutical Education*, *82*(7), 6324. doi:10.5688/ajpe6324 PMID:30323387

Saseen, J. J. (2017). ACCP clinical pharmacist competencies. *Pharmacotherapy: The Journal of Human Pharmacology and Drug Therapy*, 630-636.

Savery, J. R. (2006). Overview of Problem-based Learning: Definitions and Distinctions. *The Interdisciplinary Journal of Problem-Based Learning*, *1*(1). Advance online publication. doi:10.7771/1541-5015.1002

Sawangjit, R., Khan, T. M., & Chaiyakunapruk, N. (2017). Effectiveness of pharmacy-based needle/syringe exchange programme for people who inject drugs: A systematic review and meta-analysis. *Addiction (Abingdon, England)*. Advance online publication. doi:10.1111/add.13593 PMID:27566970

ScanBalt. (2013). *Four universities collaborate to introduce a European Masters Programme in Medicines Regulatory Affairs - Scanbalt*. https://scanbalt.org/scanbalt-news/four-universities-collaborate-introduce-european-masters-programme-medicines-regulatory-affairs/

Scannell, J. W., Blanckley, A., Boldon, H., & Warrington, B. (2012). Diagnosing the decline in pharmaceutical R&D efficiency. Nature Reviews Drug Discovery. doi:10.1038/nrd3681

Schumacher, D. J., Englander, R., & Carraccio, C. (2013). Developing the master learner: Applying learning theory to the learner, the teacher, and the learning environment. *Academic Medicine*, *88*(11), 1635–1645. doi:10.1097/ACM.0b013e3182a6e8f8 PMID:24072107

Sharma, N. (2016). Cognitive load theory and teaching in primary care. *The British Journal of General Practice*, *66*(649), 430. doi:10.3399/bjgp16X686389 PMID:27481975

Sharp, M., Bodenreider, O., & Wacholder, N. (2008). A framework for characterizing drug information sources. *AMIA ... Annual Symposium Proceedings - AMIA Symposium. AMIA Symposium*, 662–666. PMID:18999182

Shea, B. J., Reeves, B. C., Wells, G., Thuku, M., Hamel, C., Moran, J., Moher, D., Tugwell, P., Welch, V., Kristjansson, E., & Henry, D. A. (2017). AMSTAR 2: A critical appraisal tool for systematic reviews that include randomised or non-randomised studies of healthcare interventions, or both. *BMJ (Clinical Research Ed.)*, *358*, j4008. doi:10.1136/bmj.j4008 PMID:28935701

Skinner, B. F. (1961). Teaching Machines. In Cumulative Record. New York: Appleton-Century-Crofts. doi:10.1037/11324-011

Skinner, D. (2010). *Effective Teaching and Learning in Practice*. Continuum International Publishing Group.

Smith, R. (1997). *The future of healthcare systems: Information technology and consumerism will transform health care worldwide*. British Medical Journal Publishing Group.

SNS. (2016). *Registo Nacional de Estudos Clínicos (RNEC)*. https://www.rnec.pt/

SNS. (2017). *Registo Nacional de Estudos Clínicos (RNEC) – SNS*. https://www.sns.gov.pt/reforma-faq/registo-nacional-de-estudos-clinicos-rnec-6/

Soares, I. B. I.-I. T. (2020). A survey to assess the availability, implementation rate and remuneration of Pharmacist-led cognitive services in Europe. Research in Social and Administrative Pharmacy, 41-47.

Sousa Pinto, G., Bader, L., Billberg, K., Criddle, D., Duggan, C., El Bizri, L., ... Laven, A. (2019). Beating non-communicable diseases in primary health care: The contribution of pharmacists and guidance from FIP to support WHO goals. *Research in Social & Administrative Pharmacy*. Advance online publication. doi:10.1016/j.sapharm.2019.10.008 PMID:31668903

Spiegel, M., & Spencer, D. (2016). Relationality Through Literature. In R. Charon, S. Dasgupta, N. Hermann, C. Irvine, E. Marcus, E. R. Colón, ... M. Spiegel (Eds.), *The Principles and Practice of Narrative Medicine* (pp. 15–36). OUP.

Stansfield, C., Brunton, G., & Rees, R. (2014). Search wide, dig deep: Literature searching for qualitative research. An analysis of the publication formats and information sources used for four systematic reviews in public health. *Research Synthesis Methods*, *5*(2), 142–151. doi:10.1002/jrsm.1100 PMID:26052653

Sterne, J. A., Hernan, M. A., Reeves, B. C., Savovic, J., Berkman, N. D., Viswanathan, M., Henry, D., Altman, D. G., Ansari, M. T., Boutron, I., Carpenter, J. R., Chan, A.-W., Churchill, R., Deeks, J. J., Hróbjartsson, A., Kirkham, J., Jüni, P., Loke, Y. K., Pigott, T. D., ... Higgins, J. P. (2016). ROBINS-I: A tool for assessing risk of bias in non-randomised studies of interventions. *BMJ (Clinical Research Ed.)*, *355*, i4919. doi:10.1136/bmj.i4919 PMID:27733354

Strang, A. F., & Baia, P. (2016). An investigation of teaching and learning in Pharmacy Education. *American Journal of Pharmaceutical Education*, *80*(4), 59. doi:10.5688/ajpe80459 PMID:27293226

Strengthening a Workforce for Innovative Regulatory Science in Therapeutics Development. (2012). In *Strengthening a Workforce for Innovative Regulatory Science in Therapeutics Development*. doi:10.17226/13283

Strengthening Training of Academia in Regulatory Science (CSA STARS). (n.d.). Academic Press.

Sugihara, T. (2014). Current and ideal stages of pharmaceutical education. Yakugaku Zasshi. doi:10.1248/yakushi.14-00215-2

Supapaan, T., Low, B. Y., Wongpoowarak, P., Moolasarn, S., & Anderson, C. (2019). A transition from the BPharm to the PharmD degree in five selected countries. *Pharmacy Practice*, *17*(3), 1611. doi:10.18549/PharmPract.2019.3.1611 PMID:31592299

SYMPATHY Consortium. (2017). *Polypharmacy Management by 2030: a patient safety challenge*. SYMPATHY Consortium.

Taine, S. I. (1963). The Medical Literature Analysis and Retrieval System. *Bulletin of the Medical Library Association*, *51*, 157–167. PMID:13980229

Tawfik, G. M., Dila, K. A. S., Mohamed, M. Y. F., Tam, D. N. H., Kien, N. D., Ahmed, A. M., & Huy, N. T. (2019). A step by step guide for conducting a systematic review and meta-analysis with simulation data. *Tropical Medicine and Health*, *47*(1), 46. doi:10.118641182-019-0165-6 PMID:31388330

Teagarden, J. R. (2013). Well Connected: Pharmacy Education and the Humanities. *The Journal of Medical Humanities*, *34*(4), 477–480. doi:10.100710912-013-9249-1 PMID:23979798

Teagarden, J. R., Assa-Eley, M., & Nemire, R. E. (2013). Illness Performed and Imagined: An elective course using Humanities to teach student pharmacists about illness. *Currents in Pharmacy Teaching & Learning*, *5*(2), 120–128. doi:10.1016/j.cptl.2012.09.017

Thiele, R., Poiro, N., Scalzo, D., & Nemergut, E. (2010). Speed, accuracy, and confidence in Google, Ovid, PubMed, and UpToDate: Results of a randomized trial. *Postgraduate Medical Journal*, *86*(1018), 459–465. doi:10.1136/pgmj.2010.098053 PMID:20709767

Tietze, K. J. (2012). *Researching and Providing Drug Information Clinical Skills for Pharmacists* (3rd ed.). Mosby.

Timpe, E. M., Motl, S. E., & Eichner, S. F. (2006). Weekly active-learning activities in a drug information and literature evaluation course. *American Journal of Pharmaceutical Education*, *70*(3), 52. doi:10.5688/aj700352 PMID:17136173

Toklu, H. Z., & Hussain, A. (2013). The changing face of pharmacy practice and the need for a new model of pharmacy education. *Journal of Young Pharmacists*. E-Flow Medknow Publications. doi:10.1016/j.jyp.2012.09.001

Tominaga, T., Asahina, Y., Uyama, Y., & Kondo, T. (2011). Regulatory science as a bridge between science and society. *Clinical Pharmacology and Therapeutics*, *90*(1), 1–3. doi:10.1038/clpt.2011.89 PMID:21691273

Tuckman, B. W. (1965). Developmental sequence in small groups. *Psychological Bulletin*, *63*(6), 384–399. doi:10.1037/h0022100 PMID:14314073

United Nations. (2012). *Resolution adopted by the General Assembly on 12 December 2012*. Resolutions and Decisions.

United Nations. (2019). *Transforming our world: The 2030 agenda for sustainable development United Nations transforming our world: The 2030 agenda for sustainable development*. Retrieved from https://sustainabledevelopment.un.org/content/documents/21252030 Agenda for Sustainable Development web.pdf

University of Copenhagen. (2020). *European University Collaboration – University of Copenhagen*. https://mra.ku.dk/behind/pharmatrain/

van Mil, J. (2019). Seamless care, do it well or not at all. *International Journal of Clinical Pharmacy*, 1391–1393. PMID:31748966

Vanstone, M., Toledo, F., Clarke, F., Boyle, A., Giacomini, M., Swinton, M., … Cook, D. (2016). Narrative medicine and death in the ICU: word clouds as a visual legacy. *BMJ Supportive & Palliative Care*. doi:10.1136/bmjspcare-2016-001179

Vogt, E. M., & Finley, P. R. (2009). Heart of pharmacy: A course exploring the psychosocial issues of patient care. *American Journal of Pharmaceutical Education*, *73*(8), 149. Advance online publication. doi:10.5688/aj7308149 PMID:20221342

Volmer, D., Sepp, K., Raal, A., & Atkinson, J. (2019). Pharmacy Practice and Education in Estonia. *Pharmacy (Basel, Switzerland)*, *7*(3), 87. Advance online publication. doi:10.3390/pharmacy7030087 PMID:31295797

Vygotsky, L. S. (1978). *Mind in Society*. Harvard University Press.

Walton, C. A. (2006). Education and training of the drug information specialist. 1967. *The Annals of Pharmacotherapy*, *40*(2), 311–315. doi:10.1345/aph.140008 PMID:16452084

Wang, F., Troutman, W. G., Seo, T., Peak, A., & Rosenberg, J. M. (2006). Drug information education in doctor of pharmacy programs. *American Journal of Pharmaceutical Education, 70*(3), 51. doi:10.5688/aj700351 PMID:17136172

Warholak, T. L., Holdford, D. A., West, D., Debake, D. L., Bentley, J. P., Malone, D. C., & Murphy, J. E. (2011). Perspectives on educating pharmacy students about the science of safety. *American Journal of Pharmaceutical Education, 75*(7), 142. Advance online publication. doi:10.5688/ajpe757142 PMID:21969728

Watanabe, A. S., McCart, G., Shimomura, S., & Kayser, S. (1975). Systematic approach to drug information requests. *American Journal of Hospital Pharmacy, 32*(12), 1282–1285. PMID:1211401

Watson, J. B. (1930). *Behaviorism*. W. W. Norton.

Wells, G., Shea, B., O'Connell, D., Peterson, J., Welch, V., Losos, M., & Tugwell, P. (2000). *The Newcastle–Ottawa Scale (NOS) for Assessing the Quality of Non-Randomized Studies in Meta-Analysis*. Academic Press.

Whitehead, A., & Woods, A. (2016). *The Edinburgh Companion to the Critical Medical Humanities* (S. Atkinson, J. Macnaughton, & J. Richards, Eds.). Edinburgh University Press. Retrieved from http://www.jstor.org/stable/10.3366/j.ctt1bgzddd

WHO. (1948). *Constitution of WHO*. Official Records of WHO.

WHO. (1994). *The Role of the Pharmacist in the Health Care System.* Report based on a WHO meeting, Tokyo, Japan. (WHO/PHARM/94.569)

WHO. (2012). The Pursuit of Responsible Use of Medicines: Sharing and Learning from Country Experiences. *The Veterinary Record, 169*(9), 78. doi:10.1136/vr.d5420

WHO. (2019). The legal and regulatory framework for community pharmacies in the WHO European Region. Copenhagen: World Health Organization, Regional Office for Europe. License: CC BY-NC-SA 3.0 IGO.

Wiedenmayer, K., Summers, R. S., Mackie, C. A., Gous, A. G. S., Everard, M., & Tromp, D. (2006). Developing pharmacy practice - A focus on patient care. *World Health Organization, International Pharmaceutical Federation*, 87. Retrieved from http://scholar.google.com/scholar?hl=en&btnG=Search&q=intitle:Developing+pharmacy+practice+A+focus+on+patient+care#3%0Ahttp://www.who.int/iris/handle/10665/69399

Wiedenmayer, K., Summers, R. S., Mackie, C. A., Gous, A. G. S., Everard, M., Tromp, D., & Organization, W. H. (2006). *Developing pharmacy practice: a focus on patient care: handbook*. World Health Organization.

Wood, E. H., Morrison, J. L., & Oppenheimer, P. R. (1990). Drug information skills for pharmacy students: Curriculum integration. *Bulletin of the Medical Library Association, 78*(1), 8–14. PMID:2295022

World Health Organisation. (2017). *WHO | What is universal coverage?* Health Financing for Universal Coverage.

World Health Organization (WHO). (1996). *Good pharmacy practice (GPP) in community and hospital pharmacy settings* [WHO/PHARM/DAP/96.1]. WHO.

World Health Organization (WHO). (1997). The role of the pharmacist in the health care system, preparing the future pharmacist: curricular development: report of a third WHO Consultative Group on the Role of the Pharmacist. World Health Organization.

World Health Organization. (1997). *The Role of the Pharmacist in the Health Care System - Preparing the future pharmacist: curricular development*. Retrieved from https://apps.who.int/medicinedocs/pdf/whozip32e/whozip32e.pdf

World Health Organization. (2007). Everybody business: strengthening health systems to improve health outcomes: WHO's framework for action. *Production*.

World Health Organization. (2013). *Arguing for Universal Health Coverage*. World Health Organization. doi:10.1016/j.memsci.2011.12.046

World Medical Association. (1999). Statement on the Working Relationship between Physicians and Pharmacists in Medicinal Therapy. 51st World Medical Assembly, Tel Aviv, Israel.

Wright, E. A., Brown, B., Gettig, J., Martello, J. L., McClendon, K. S., Smith, K. M., Teeters, J., Ulbrich, T. R., Wegrzyn, N., & Bradley-Baker, L. R. (2014). Teaching and learning curriculum programs: Recommendations for postgraduate pharmacy experiences in education. *American Journal of Health-System Pharmacy*, *71*(15), 1292–1302. doi:10.2146/ajhp130657 PMID:25027537

Yang, N., Xiao, H., Cao, Y., Li, S., Yan, H., & Wang, Y. (2018). Does narrative medicine education improve nursing students' empathic abilities and academic achievement? A randomised controlled trial. *The Journal of International Medical Research*, *46*(8), 3306–3317. doi:10.1177/0300060518781476 PMID:29976109

Young, T., Rohwer, A., Volmink, J., & Clarke, M. (2014). What are the effects of teaching evidence-based health care (EBHC)? Overview of systematic reviews. *PLoS One*, *9*(1), e86706. doi:10.1371/journal.pone.0086706 PMID:24489771

Zimmermann, M. (2013). Integrating medical humanities into a pharmaceutical care seminar on dementia. *American Journal of Pharmaceutical Education*, *77*(1), 1–8. doi:10.5688/ajpe77116 PMID:23459365

About the Contributors

Isabel Vitória Figueiredo is an Associate Professor with aggregation at Group of Pharmacology and Pharmaceutical Care / Faculty of Pharmacy, University of Coimbra. Her main research areas are Pharmacology and Pharmacotherapy. She authored and/or co-authored more than 50 articles in national/international journals. She supervised 11 Ph.D. and 20 Master's theses. She integrates and/or coordinates diverse research groups/units. Among others, she integrates the Scientific Council of the Institute of Nuclear Sciences Applied to Health, and she is a founding member of the Portuguese Association of Experimental Pathology and the Portuguese Society of Sciences in Laboratory Animals and current President of the Board. ORCiD identifier: https://orcid.org/0000-0003-0127-4575.

Afonso Miguel Cavaco holds an MSc in Community Pharmacy (Faculty of Pharmacy, University of Lisbon - FFUL) and a Ph.D. in Pharmacy Practice and Policy (The School of Pharmacy, UCL). He was a postdoctoral Fulbright fellow in Health Communication (Johns Hopkins University, USA). Presently he is Associate Professor at FFUL, responsible for undergraduate and postgraduate courses in Social Pharmacy and Health Communication. He has more than 65 original peer-reviewed papers in indexed journals, amongst other communications on the use of medicines and social pharmacy. His main research interests are on patient-professionals interactions, health written information and patient safety. ORCiD identifier: https://orcid.org/0000-0001-8466-0484.

* * *

Maria José de Almeida is an Emeritus Professor at the Physics Department of the Faculty of Sciences and Technology of the University of Coimbra (UC). She was proponent, coordinator and the leading professor of both Bologna master's degree for Physics and Chemistry Teachers Education and of the Ph.D. on Sciences Teaching of UC. She taught Physics Didactics and oriented Physics Educational Projects. For several years, she co-coached yearly in-School practice stages for Physics Teacher

Students, together with a School partner, within University-School Partnerships for Teacher Education and Educational Research in Practice. ORCiD identifier: https://orcid.org/0000-0002-5814-968X.

Filipa Alves da Costa is an Associate Professor at Instituto Universitário Egas Moniz and Invited Professor at the Faculty of Pharmacy, University of Lisbon (FFUL). She is associated with CiiEM and iMED research centers. Filipa works for the National Oncology Register as responsible for the effectiveness area. She holds an MSc in Community Pharmacy (FFUL) and a Ph.D. in Pharmacy Practice and Policy (University College of London). She is actively involved in various international organizations, namely the European Society of Clinical Pharmacy (vice-chair of education committee), International Pharmaceutical Federation (ExCo of Social and Administrative Pharmacy Section), International Pharmacists for Anticoagulation Care Taskforce (board member) and Pharmaceutical Care Network Europe (chair in 2007). ORCiD identifier: https://orcid.org/0000-0003-0562-2514.

Cecilia Beecher Martins is Invited Assistant Professor in the English Studies Department at the School of Arts & Humanities, where she teaches Canadian literature, film and literary analysis and English language University of Lisbon, as well as semiotics of cinema in a variety of Narrative Medicine/Medical Humanities teaching modules at the School of Arts & Humanities, the Medical Faculty and the Nursing School of the University of Lisbon. She is a researcher at ULICES (the University of Lisbon Centre for English Studies) where she belongs to the American Studies Research Group and the Medical Humanities Research Project. She has published essays and chapters as well as co-edited books and a special edition of a research journal on Narrative Medicine and Film Studies. ORCiD identifier: https://orcid.org/0000-0003-3206-5856.

Helena H. Borba Ph.D. in Pharmaceutical Sciences, Federal University of Paraná (Brazil). Master's Degree in collaboration with the Private Universität für Gesundheitswissenschaften, Medizinische Informatik und Technik (Austria). Professor of Pharmaceutical Care subject in the Department of Pharmacy, Federal University of Paraná (Brazil). Postdoctoral researcher and member of the Group of Studies in Health-Technology Assessment (GEATS). Research interests: health-technology assessment, pharmacoeconomic modeling, evidence synthesis. ORCiD identifier: https://orcid.org/0000-0001-9723-584X.

Maria de Jesus Cabral holds a PhD in Modern Literature and Languages, specialization in French Literature, with a thesis on Mallarmé and Maeterlinck's Theatre (Catholic University of Portugal, 2005), published by Eds Rodopi. From

2007 to 2011, she carried out post-doctoral research in Portuguese Poetic Theatre (between Eugénio de Castro and Fernando Pessoa) at the University of Coimbra. Between 1994 and 2015, she was a full-time Professor of French and Francophone Literature at the Catholic University of Portugal and an invited Professor at the University of Coimbra; today, she is a full Researcher and invited Professor at FLUL. Her research focuses mainly on Symbolist Poetry from a comparative and interdisciplinary perspective, on its relationship with theatre, literary reading and translation. She develops research and education programs in Medical Humanities within the Project "Medicine Narrative" (ULICES/CEAUL), addressing more specifically the relationship between theatre and medicine from a conceptual and methodological perspective. She is the author of Mallarmé hors frontières (2007) and has published several original papers in indexed scientific journals and collective works, among which are: Lumières de Camus (2012); Lire, de près, de loin. Close Vs Distant reading (2014); Contar (com) a Medicina (2015, reed. 2016); Maux écrits, mots vécus: traitements littéraires de la maladie (2015); Exotopies de Barthes (2016); Santé et Bien-être à l'épreuve de la Littérature (2017). ORCiD identifier: https://orcid.org/0000-0002-0736-3846.

Teresa Casal is an Assistant Professor at the School of Arts and Humanities, University of Lisbon, and a researcher at the University of Lisbon Centre for Lisbon Studies (ULICES). Her current research in Irish Studies and Medical Humanities focuses on how contemporary narrative fiction and creative non-fiction are used to make sense of life, loss and illness. She has co-edited the literary anthology Contar (com) a Medicina (2015; 2016; 2018), Beyond Diagnosis: Relating Person to Patient, Patient to Person (2014), and Revisitar o Mito / Myths Revisited (2015). She is also a literary translator. ORCiD identifier: https://orcid.org/0000-0002-6741-406X.

Fernando Fernandez-Llimos holds a Ph.D. in Pharmacy, University of Granada (Spain). Professor at the Laboratory of Pharmacology, Department of Drug Sciences, Faculty of Pharmacy, University of Porto (Portugal). Member of the Health Information Systems & Electronic Health Records (HIS-EHR) group of the Center for Health Technology and Services Research (CINTESIS), University of Porto. Editor-in-Chief of Pharmacy Practice. Research interests: information for healthcare professionals, pharmaceutical clinical services, evidence synthesis, epidemiologic and biostatistical methods. ORCiD identifier: https://orcid.org/0000-0002-8529-9595.

Maria-Eduardo Figueira is a Professor of Bromatology at the Faculty of Pharmacy of the University of Lisbon (Portugal) and Coordinator of the master's degree in food quality and health in the same Faculty. She is a researcher at the Pharmacological & Regulatory Research Group at iMed.ULisboa with research interest in the study of the role of some foods in the prevention of chronic diseases. Additionally, she is an assessor for the Directorate General for Food and Veterinary and member of the National Observatory of Emerging Risks of the Authority for Food and Economic Security (ASAE). ORCID ID: 0000-0002-1561-6858

Nélia Gouveia holds a PhD in Clinical Research (Epidemiology - NMS|FCM) and integrates the Rheumatic Diseases Group of CEDOC, NMS|FCM, as Clinical Researcher. She is also the Coordinator of the Master Course of Management of Clinical Research (MEGIC) in NMS|FCM, provided by Universidade NOVA and Universidade de Aveiro. As a professor, beyond MEGIC, Nélia collaborates at Doctoral Programme in Medicine and PhD Programme in Mechanisms of Disease and Regenerative Medicine of NMS|FCM. Moreover, she coordinates the Clinical Trial Unit Project of NOVA, named NOVA CRU, supporting independent clinical studies. Nélia Gouveia is author and co-author of more than 20 scientific articles published in national and international peer-review journals. She wan some national prizes of clinical research (Prémio Dor Grunenthal 2015, as 1st author and Grande Prémio Bial da Medicina 2017, as 3rd author). ORCiD identifier: https://orcid.org/0000-0003-4977-0367.

Mara Pereira Guerreiro is an Invited Professor, R&D Project Leader, and entrepreneur pharmacist. She is driven by positively impact people's lives through interdisciplinary research and by teaching tomorrow's and today's health care professionals. In addition to gaining an array of research skills in her PhD and post-doctoral work, Mara embraced state-of-the-art approaches in digital technology, such as co-production and open innovation. Her key competences include research projects funding, leadership & management, science communication & dissemination, plus digital transformation of teaching and learning in higher education for efficiency and sustainability gains. She is the leader of national and European funded projects in digital technology (https://vaselfcare.rd.ciencias.ulisboa.pt and https://www.train4health.eu). Her communication and dissemination efforts include book editing, book chapters, and, overall, more than 150 papers and presentations in scientific events, including plenary sessions by invitation, posters, oral communications, and workshops. She implemented and evaluated innovative pedagogical practices with the aid of digital technology, such as "team-based learning", "flipped classroom", online summative assessment, and serious games. She was distinguished as a "fellow" by the European Society of Clinical Pharmacy (2018), and her work was awarded in several scientific events. Her international profile is also evidenced by her role in governing bodies of European scientific associations and by the organisation of international scientific events in her interest areas. Mara's personal values are hard work, initiative, creativity, commitment, integrity, and leading by example. She is passionate about acquiring new knowledge and skills and enjoys challenging herself to expand her comfort zone. - ORCiD identifier https://orcid.org/0000-0001-8192-6080.

Maria Teresa Herdeiro Teresa Herdeiro is a Pharmacist with a PhD in Public Health, a Master in Pharmaceutical Sciences and a Master in Food Science and Engineering. She is also a Regulatory Affairs Specialist by Portuguese Pharmacist College. Auxiliar Professor and also the Coordinator of the Master Course of Management of Clinical Research (MEGIC) at Aveiro University (UA), provided by UA and Universidade NOVA. She is a principal investigator in iBiMED/UA and her main research interests are public health, pharmacoepidemiology, pharmacovigilance, regulatory sciences. In 2012, she received the award for Scientific Research Professor Maria Odette Santos Ferreira, in 2016 the award for Public Health and Clinic Epidemiology by Medical Science Lisbon Society. She is an editor and reviewer of several scientific journals, a member of ENCePP Steering Group-EMA. She has published 5 chapters of books and has authored and/or co-authored more than 50 papers in peer-review scientific journals. She supervised 5 PhD and 30 masters. She is an Investigator in several projects financed by FCT, CNPq, QREN, FIS and MC Member-PT for a COST Action. https://orcid.org/0000-0002-0500-4049.

Maria Margarida Caramona is an Emeritus Professor at the Group of Pharmacology and Pharmaceutical Care, at Faculty of Pharmacy of the Coimbra University, Portugal (UC). She teaches courses of pharmacology, pharmacotherapy, clinical pharmacy, pharmaceutical care and was responsible for training students in the community and the hospital pharmacies during pre-graduate career. At the present, she works in continuous education programs in cooperation with the Portuguese Pharmaceutical Society (Ordem dos Farmacêuticos) and is the coordinator of a Platform teaching/profession to promote the relationship between the pharmacy university teachers and the pharmaceutical professionals. ORCiD identifier: https://orcid.org/0000-0003-1950-9360.

Catarina Martins Pires holds a MPharm degree in Pharmaceutical Sciences. Presently works as a community pharmacist.

Antonio M. Mendes Pharmacist at the Clinical Hospital (HC) of Curitiba and Ph.D. student in Pharmaceutical Sciences, Federal University of Paraná (Brazil). Master's Degree in Internal Medicine (Federal University of Paraná, Brazil). Specialist in Clinical and Hospital Care of the adult and elderly (HC - Brazil). Research interests: health-technology assessment, pharmaceutical clinical services, epidemiologic and biostatistical methods, bibliometrics. ORCiD identifier: https://orcid.org/0000-0002-5752-349X.

Ema Paulino is a community pharmacist at her own pharmacy in Portugal. Since October 2019, Ema is General Manager and Scientific Coordinator at Ezfy. She is a member of the National Board of the Portuguese Pharmaceutical Society (Ordem dos Farmacêuticos). Ema is currently the Professional Secretary of the International Pharmaceutical Federation and a member of its Bureau, having previously been Chairperson and Project Coordinator of the Young Pharmacists' Group, a member of the FIP Programme Committee, and Secretary of the Community Pharmacy Section. Ema is also Chairperson of the Pharmaceutical Care Network Europe. ORCiD identifier: https://orcid.org/0000-0002-4087-375X.

Margarida Pinto Dias holds a MPharm degree in Pharmaceutical Sciences. Presently works as a community pharmacist.

Roberto Pontarolo holds a Ph.D. in Sciences – Biochemistry, from the Federal University of Paraná (Brazil). Professor at the Pharmacy Department and coordinator of the Postgraduate Research Program in Pharmaceutical Care, Federal University of Paraná (Brazil). Leader of the research Center of Biopharmacy (CEB) and Group of Studies in Health-Technology Assessment (GEATS). Member of the advisory board of the Brazilian Regulatory Agency (ANVISA), of the Brazilian Network of Health-Technology Assessment (REBRATS) and the National Institute of Science and Technology for Pharmaceutical Innovation (INCT-IF). Research interests: bioanalytical method validation, characterization of pharmaceutical products, health technology assessment. ORCiD identifier: https://orcid.org/0000-0002-7049-4363.

João Rocha is a Professor of Pharmacology, Immunopharmacology & Pharmacotherapy at the Faculty of Pharmacy - University of Lisbon (Portugal) and a researcher at the Pharmacological & Regulatory Research Group at iMed.ULisboa. His research interests involve experimental models of local and systemic inflammation. Additionally, he is a non-clinical assessor for the National Authority for Medicines and Health Products and a pharmaceutical and toxicological assessor for the Directorate-General for Food and Veterinary. He is also a member of the Council for Cooperation of the Professional Board of Pharmacists with the responsibility of implementing advanced education programs in Portuguese Speaking Countries. ORCiD identifier: https://orcid.org/0000-0002-0303-8085.

Fátima Roque is a pharmacist with PhD in Pharmaceutical Sciences and with Master in Drug Technology. She is also a Regulatory Affairs Specialist by Portuguese Pharmacist College. Adjunct Professor at Health Sciences School of Polytechnic

Institute of Guarda. She is an investigator in the Center of Health Sciences (CICS/UBI), and her main research interests are pharmacotherapy, pharmacoepidemiology and public health. She is a guest editor (2 indexed International Journals) and reviewer of several scientific journals. She received the Clinical Epidemiology Prize, awarded by the Society of Medical Sciences of Lisbon, in 2016. She has published 3 chapters of books and is authored and/or co-authored more than 30 papers in peer-review scientific journals. She is a principal investigator for two projects funded by FCT in the field of polymedication in the elderly, the MedElderly project and the APIMedOlder project. She is also a researcher in 2 other projects in the area of bacterial resistance (eHealthResp) and one in the field of pharmaceutical development (DermoBio), funded by FCT. ORCiD identifier: https://orcid.org/0000-0003-0169-3788.

Mariana Rosa holds a master's degree in Pharmaceutical Sciences from the Faculty of Health Sciences - University of Beira Interior. After finishing her studies, she collaborated with an NGO in Mozambique as a volunteer at a Nutrition Care Centre, developing the area of health promotion. From 2013 to 2019, she has worked as a project manager at Farmácias Holon, contributing to the development and implementation of new services at the community pharmacy level. Since October 2019, she is Solution Designer at Ezfy, where she designs Patient Support Programs which engage community pharmacists.

Bruno Sepodes is a Professor of Pharmacology and Pharmacotherapy at the Faculty of Pharmacy of the University of Lisbon (Portugal), working closely with professionals in order to bridge Academy and Pharmacy Practice. He is a Senior Non-Clinical Expert for the Portuguese National Authority for Medicines and Health Products and became a member of the European Medicines Agency's Committee for Orphan Medicinal Products (COMP) in 2008, serving for two mandates as Chairperson of this Committee (2012-2018). Additionally, Bruno is also a member and Vice-Chair of the European Medicines Agency's Committee for Human Medicinal Products (CHMP) and a member of the Committee of Advanced Therapies (CAT). ORCiD identifier: https://orcid.org/0000-0002-2761-0955.

Fernanda S. Tonin holds a PhD in Pharmacy from the Federal University of Paraná (Brazil) and University of Lisbon (Portugal). Master's Degree in Pharmaceutical Sciences, Federal University of Paraná (Brazil). Postgraduate Visiting Researcher at the University of Technology Sydney (Australia). Member of the Group of Studies in Health-Technology Assessment (GEATS). Consultant of healthcare products and services providing support for evidence synthesis, clinical research and medical writing. Research interests: health-technology assessment, decision-analytic modeling, pharmacoeconomic assessment, epidemiologic and biostatistical methods. ORCiD identifier: https://orcid.org/0000-0003-4262-8608.

Index

L

M

N

P

R

S

T

U

W

www.ingramcontent.com/pod-product-compliance
Lightning Source LLC
LaVergne TN
LVHW081520300926
849161LV00006B/1235
* 9 7 8 1 7 9 9 8 4 4 8 6 0 *